ANGIOGRAPHY OF POSTERIOR FOSSA TUMORS

ANGIOGRAPHY OF POSTERIOR FOSSA TUMORS

Samuel M. Wolpert, M.B.B.Ch., D.M.R.D.

Professor of Radiology
Tufts University School of Medicine
and Chief of Neuroradiology
Tufts-New England Medical Center Hospital
Boston, Massachusetts

With a chapter on
**Clinical and Pathological Aspects
of Posterior Fossa Tumors**

BENNETT M. STEIN, M.D.C.M., F.A.C.S.

Professor and Chairman of Neurological Surgery
Tufts-New England Medical Center Hospital
Boston, Massachusetts

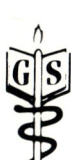

GRUNE & STRATTON

A Subsidiary of Harcourt Brace Jovanovich, Publishers
New York   San Francisco   London

Library of Congress Cataloging in Publication Data
Wolpert, Samuel M
 Angiography of posterior fossa tumors.

 Bibliography : p.
 Includes index.
 1. Brain—Tumors—Diagnosis. 2. Brain—Blood vessels—Radiography. 3. Cranial fossa, Posterior.
I. Stein, Bennett M. II. Title.
RC280.B7W63   616.9'92'81   75-37783
ISBN 0-8089-0924-X

© *1976 by Grune & Stratton, Inc.*
All rights reserved. No part of this publication
may be reproduced or transmitted in any form or
by any means, electronic or mechanical, including
photocopy, recording, or any information storage
and retrieval system, without permission in
writing from the publisher.

Grune & Stratton, Inc.
111 Fifth Avenue
New York, New York 10003

Library of Congress Catalog Card Number 75-37783
International Standard Book Number 0-8089-0924-X
Printed in the United States of America

To Cynthia
David, Michelle, and Steven

CONTENTS

Acknowledgments
Preface

1. Historical Aspects of Vertebral Angiography — 1
2. Techniques of Vertebral Angiography — 4
   Angiographic Technique
   Complications
   Radiographic Technique
   Subtraction
   Angiotomography
3. Clinical and Pathological Aspects of Posterior Fossa Tumors — 20
   Syndromes
   Pathology
   Surgical Considerations
4. Normal Angiographic Anatomy of Posterior Fossa — 31
   Vertebral Artery
   Basilar Artery
   Meningeal Arteries
   Cervicovertebral Veins
   Posterior Fossa Veins
   Supratentorial Veins
5. Prepontine and Cerebellopontine Angle Tumors — 91
   Retrocerebellar Extra-axial Tumors
6. Pontine and Mesencephalic Tumors — 115
   Quadrigeminal Plate Tumors
7. Fourth Ventricle Tumors — 129
8. Vermian and Hemispheric Tumors — 146
   Inferior Vermian and Inferior Hemispheric Tumors
   Tonsillar Herniation
   Superior Vermian and Superior Hemispheric Tumors
9. Differential Diagnosis of Posterior Fossa Tumors — 176
   Acoustic Neurinomas
   Meningiomas
   Fifth Nerve Neurinomas
   Hemangioblastomas

Glomus Jugulare Tumors
Miscellaneous Tumors

Index 181

ACKNOWLEDGMENTS

I am indebted to many people for this book, particularly the neuroradiology team at Tufts-New England Medical Center, who have provided the quality of angiographic dedication we have considered necessary. Mrs. Eileen Galvin, R.N., and Mr. Ted Gruber, R.T., with aid from their respective nursing and technician colleagues, have helped immeasurably. Mr. Serge Kajko was instrumental in designing the photographic light box and subsequently provided the subtraction studies necessary for identification of the posterior fossa vessels. The illustrations are the work of Mr. Robert Ulrich, medical artist.

A book like this could never be written without editorial, secretarial, and typographical help. To acknowledge these attributes in one person is part of the thanks made to the contribution of Mrs. Jeannie Leary. I am indeed fortunate to have had her help through the interminable months when the final text seemed never to appear.

A special vote of thanks is given to E. R. Squibb & Sons, Inc., whose generous gift helped make it possible to publish the color line diagrams.

PREFACE

The recent dramatic appearance of computerized axial tomography brings into high relief questions about the future utilization of vertebral angiography in the evaluation of posterior fossa tumors. To quote Di Chiro (1974) in an editorial, "According to latter day Cassandras, pneumoencephalography is in its last throes, and the fate of radionuclide brain scanning is not much brighter. . . . Cerebral angiography fares a little better, but only in reference to certain specific conditions, as berry aneurysms." Di Chiro goes on to caution these soothsayers and pleads for temperization and the avoidance of haste before considering that neuroradiology has died and with it the old methodologies.*

Preliminary results have demonstrated that computerized tomography can identify the majority of posterior fossa tumors above a minimal size. Certain problems presented by the complex configuration of the adjacent bone and the presence of air-containing cavities need to be overcome, however. Furthermore, many neurosurgeons still require an angiographic road map before tackling a posterior fossa tumor suspect. This is especially applicable to prepontine masses.

The ease of performance and diagnosis of computerized tomographic scanning stands in sharp contrast to the difficulties of performance and diagnosis of posterior fossa angiography. Apart from the skills necessary to safely carry out a posterior angiogram, the neophyte physician in radiology, neurology, or neurosurgery, on being confronted by a posterior fossa angiogram, is faced with a bewildering array of arteries and veins. The perplexity of the neuroanatomy of the vessels has dismayed all but the most intrepid. Like any other vascular system in the body, however, these vessels bear a consistent relationship to normal pontine and cerebellar structures. An understanding of these anatomical relationships is all-important and needs to be firmly established before the pathological angiogram can be interpreted.

To assist the reader in developing the anatomical background necessary to correlate the relationship of the major vessels to the pons, fourth ventricle, and cerebellum, a series of colored line diagrams has been developed where the relationships are exaggerated and emphasized. A similar series of colored line diagrams stresses the pathological displacements. In approaching this book, the reader should constantly and repetitively refer to the line diagrams at the beginning of Chapter 4 and view them in conjunction with the angiograms. In this manner, the "pattern" of the normal vertebral angiogram should be consolidated in the reader's eye, allowing him to immediately recognize the abnormal.

*Di Chiro G: Of *CAT* and other beasts (editorial). Amer J Roentgenol 122:659, 1974.

Preface

The future is uncertain—our diagnostic methodologies are changing, and the ultimate role of posterior fossa angiography, where computerized tomography is available, is unclear. The tomographic machines are, however, expensive, and until such time as the manufacturers can reduce the cost and make the machines more readily available, angiography will continuc to play its dominant role in the elucidation of posterior fossa tumors.

1
Historical Aspects of Vertebral Angiography

Forty years have passed since Moniz and Alves[1] reported on the successful, but accidental, demonstration of the posterior fossa circulation after an injection of radiopaque contrast agent into the common carotid artery.[2] The opacification of the posterior fossa was obtained fortuitously by reflux of the contrast agent into the subclavian artery. As a result of the success of Moniz and Alves, during the subsequent two decades there were attempts to improve the original method by directly injecting contrast agent into the subclavian artery, either percutaneously or after open surgery.[3,4]

Direct vertebral puncture was initially achieved after open surgery to identify the vessel.[5] In 1940, however, Takahashi reported on the successful percutaneous puncture of the vertebral artery in the neck with an endhole needle,[6] and for a number of years, this was the preferred method in many hospital centers.[7,8,9] The development of a needle with a plugged endhole but an open sidehole, by Sheldon in 1956, greatly facilitated the technique of percutaneous puncture of the artery.[10]

A milestone in the development of vertebral angiography was reached in 1947 when Radner, after surgically exposing the radial artery, inserted a urethral catheter under fluoroscopic control and injected 36 percent Diotrast® after the catheter had entered the vertebral artery.[11]

In subsequent years, indirect methods of opacifying the vertebral artery were developed, utilizing either percutaneous subclavian punctures or surgical exposures of the femoral artery and the threading of catheters up the aorta into the subclavian artery.

In 1953, Seldinger described his revolutionary method of percutaneous puncture of the femoral artery with replacement of the needle and insertion of a catheter.[12] The adaptation of this technique to catheterization of the subclavian artery and routine visualization of the vertebral artery was not immediately appreciated. In fact, in 1956, Lindgren reported on a method of catheterization of the subclavian artery after percutaneous puncture of the femoral artery with a thick cannula through which a polyethylene catheter was inserted.[13] In 1958, however, Bonte, Riff, and Spy reported on the successful selective catheterization of the left vertebral artery by Seldinger's method after a transfemoral approach.[14] Transaxillary catheterization of the vertebral artery was developed by Roy, Jutras, and Longtin in 1961[15] and subsequently found to be very useful in patients with marked atherosclerosis of the iliac arteries and aorta.[16,17] Since then, many angiographers have adopted Seldinger's method, and it has become firmly established in many hospitals as the preferred method of vertebral angiography.

Brachial angiography with the retrograde injection of contrast agent after surgical exposure of the brachial artery was described as an alternative method of vertebral angiography in 1955 by Gould, Peyton, and French.[18] Percutaneous brachial angiography to visualize the vertebral artery after the insertion of a catheter utilizing the Seldinger technique was reported by Pygott and Hutton in 1959.[19] Sutton, in 1959, in a letter to the editor of the British Journal of Radiology, stated that he had used percutaneous brachial catheterization since mid-1956.[20] He referred to the tendency of the artery to go into spasm after catheterization. Credit for the first reported *percutaneous* retrograde brachial angiogram with a pressure injector, but without catheter insertion, should be given to Marshall and Ling in 1963.[21] Today, this method is probably the most widely used method of obtaining opacification of the posterior fossa circulation.

REFERENCES

1. Moniz E, Alves A: L'importance diagnostique de l'artériographie de la fossa postérieure. Rev Neurol 40:91, 1933
2. Schechter MM, deGutiérrez-Mahoney CG: The evolution of vertebral angiography. Neuroradiology 5:157, 1973
3. Moniz E, Pinto A, Alves A: Artériographie du cervelet et des autres organes de la fosse postérieure. Bull Acad de Med, Paris 109:758, 1933
4. Shimidzu K: Beiträge zur arteriographie des Gehirns-einfache percutane methode. Arch f Klin Chir 188:295, 1937
5. Sjövist O: Arteriographische Darstellung der Gefässe der hinteren Schädelgrube. Chirurg 10:377, 1938
6. Takahashi K: Die Percutane Arteriographie der Arteria vertebralis und ihrer Versorgungsgebiete. Arch Psychiatr Nervenkr 111:373, 1940
7. Sugar O, Holden LB, Powell CB: Vertebral angiography. Am J Roentgenol 61:166, 1949

Historical Aspects of Vertebral Angiography

8. Lindgren E: Percutaneous angiography of the vertebral artery. Acta Radiol 33:389, 1950
9. Sutton D, Hoare RD: Percutaneous vertebral arteriography. Br J Radiol 24:589, 1951
10. Sheldon P: Special needle for percutaneous vertebral angiography. Br J Radiol 29:231, 1956
11. Radner S: Intracranial angiography via the vertebral artery. Preliminary report of a new technique. Acta Radiol 28:838, 1947
12. Seldinger SI: Catheter replacement of needle in percutaneous arteriography. A new technique. Acta Radiol 39:368, 1953
13. Lindgren E: Another method of vertebral angiography. Acta Radiol 46:257, 1956
14. Bonte G, Riff G, Spy E: Angiographie vértebrale par cathétérisme rétrograde fémoral. Acta Radiol 50:67, 1958
15. Roy P, Jutras A, Longtin M: Extra large field angiography: technique and results. J Can Assoc Radiol 12:27, 1961
16. Hanafee W: Axillary artery approach to carotid, vertebral, abdominal aorta, and coronary angiography. Radiology 81:559, 1963
17. Newton TH: The axillary artery approach to arteriography of the aorta and its branches. Am J Roentgenol 89:275, 1963
18. Gould PL, Peyton WT, French LA: Vertebral angiography by retrograde injection of the brachial artery. J Neurosurg 12:369, 1955
19. Pygott F, Hutton CF: Vertebral arteriography by percutaneous brachial artery catheterisation. Br J Radiol 32:114, 1959
20. Sutton D: Vertebral arteriography by percutaneous brachial artery catheterisation. Br J Radiol 32:283, 1959
21. Marshall TR, Ling JT: Direct percutaneous non-catheter left and right brachial angiography (left panarteriography—right cerebral angiography). Radiology 50:258, 1963

2
Techniques of Vertebral Angiography

ANGIOGRAPHIC TECHNIQUE

The technique of vertebral angiography is all important and needs the application of meticulous attention to detail at all phases of the procedure. The technique as developed and performed at this hospital has provided us with satisfactory results. This is not to say that in other institutions different techniques will not provide as satisfactory a standard. Whatever techniques are used, however, vertebral angiography must be a routine procedure and be carried out under the care of a trained and experienced team of physicians, nurses, and technicians.

On the day preceding the angiogram, the procedure should be carefully explained to the patient. A cooperative patient makes the technicians', nurses', and physicians' tasks much easier and leads to a shorter procedure with less risk of complications. The patient should have no fluid or food intake for at least 4 hours prior to the procedure.

On arrival in the neuroradiology suite, the patient should be alert but sedated. It is vitally important to monitor the patient throughout the study, and with light sedation and local anesthesia, the patient's state of consciousness, speech, visual acuity, limb strength, etc., can be evaluated.[1] The average adult receives 100 mg of Nembutal (sodium pentobarbitol) and 0.4 mg Atropine (atropine sulfate) intramuscularly 45 minutes before the procedure. If the patient is still anxious on arrival in the suite, 5 to 10 mg of Valium (diazepam) intramuscularly is given as well.

Vertebral angiography can be carried out in infants as young as the

Table 2-1
Dosage Schedule for Children

Age (years)	M.C.P.* (cc/kilo)	Atropine Sulfate (mg)
0–1	0.05	0.1
1–5	0.1	0.2
6–10	0.1	0.3

*Never to exceed 2.0 cc.

newborn. In infants and children, we use a sedative cocktail (M.C.P.) containing 25 mg Demerol (meperidine hydrochloride), 6.25 mg Thorazine (chlorpromazine), and 6.25 mg Phenergan (promethazine hydrochloride) per cc. The dosage schedule is set out in Table 2-1. The premedication is given at least 1 hour before the procedure. If the sedation is insufficient, secobarbital is added at a dose of 2.5 mg/kg.

Selective catheterization of the vertebral artery by the Seldinger technique is utilized for all patients up to the age of 50. Above this age, selective catheterization is often carried out, but with greater reluctance. If, however, the vertebral artery can be entered with the minimum of catheter manipulation, selective catheterization can be carried out. In the presence of atherosclerotic vascular disease at any age, *selective catherization is not attempted under any circumstances*. A transfemoral approach is favored whenever possible.

There are many different types of catheters available today for arterial catheterization. The ideal catheter should have a thin wall so that the selected volume of contrast agent can be introduced through a catheter with the smallest outside diameter. The catheter should be moderately radiopaque, soft and atraumatic, and have sufficient rigidity to achieve good torque control. A catheter with all the above attributes is not currently available, and the selection of a catheter material is, therefore, usually a compromise. The catheter material favored by the author for selective vertebral angiography in different age groups is set out in Table 2-2.

In patients below the age of 30, no shaping of the catheter is necessary, since a straight catheter will enter the left vertebral artery with minimal manipulation. After the age of 30, the catheter usually has to be shaped over steam. A gentle S-shaped curve is usually adequate to catheterize the subclavian and subsequently the vertebral artery.

It is most important to assess the caliber of the vertebral artery under fluoroscopic control prior to selective vertebral artery catheterization. If the orifice of the vertebral artery is not stenosed and the diameter of the vertebral artery is at least twice as large as the diameter of the catheter, a guide wire is gently inserted into the vertebral artery through the catheter. The catheter is then threaded up over the guide wire. On withdrawal of the wire, an immediate

Table 2-2
Needle and Catheter Dimensions for Different Age Groups

Age (years)	Needle	Guide Wire (Inches)	Catheter Inches I.D.	Catheter Inches O.D.	Catheter Mm I.D.	Catheter Mm O.D.	Description
Newborn–1	20G Potts Cournand thin wall	0.021	0.025	0.038	0.64	1.00	0.025F*
1–7	19G Potts Cournand thin wall	0.025	0.037	0.048	0.94	1.23	0.037F*
8 and older	18G Arterial thin wall	0.035	0.045	0.065	1.16	1.67	0.045H*

*Becton-Dickinson Company.

backflow of blood through the catheter must occur. If there is no backflow, the catheter must be withdrawn until backflow does occur. If there is a good backflow of blood, a test injection of approximately 1 to 2 cc of contrast agent is made under fluoroscopy. The contrast agent must immediately be swept away from the catheter tip by the flow of blood surrounding the catheter. If this does not occur, the catheter must be withdrawn at once.

Because the left vertebral artery is easier to catheterize than the right and also, in most cases, is equal to or larger than the right in caliber, initial attempts at vertebral catheterization are made on the left side. If the left vertebral artery is small, an attempt at right vertebral catheterization should be made. With the use of an appropriately shaped catheter and a floppy tip guide wire, the innominate artery is catheterized. The catheter is then threaded into the right subclavian artery. The identification of the right vertebral artery and precautions prior to catheterizing the artery are the same as on the left side.

To obtain reflux of contrast agent down the opposite vertebral artery, it is advisable to thread the catheter up to approximately the level of the fourth cervical vertebra. If under fluoroscopy, the artery is seen to be tortuous or narrow, this maneuver must not be attempted.

The technique of saline perfusion of the catheter is of major importance. The perfusing saline solution contains heparin in a concentration of 2000 units/500 cc of saline. The system is closed (without access to the room air) so that there is no chance of cotton fibers or talc being introduced into the saline. Two syringes are used for saline perfusion of the catheter. With the first syringe, blood and any thrombi that may be present are aspirated from the catheter and *discarded*. With the second syringe, heparinized-saline is perfused. This two-syringe maneuver is repeated approximately every minute.

The contrast agent for injection is also incorporated in a closed system. The injection of contrast for the angiographic series is made with a pressure injector to obtain reproducible results. Rarely is 6 cc exceeded, and the delivery time is 1 second. For infants and children, correspondingly smaller injections are made (Table 2-3). Renografin 60 (meglumine diatrizoate)* is our contrast agent of choice. Conray 60 (meglumine iothalamate)† is favored by some angiographers. *Immediately after the injection of contrast agent, the catheter is withdrawn from the vertebral artery.* This rule is always adhered to. Its purpose is twofold. First, it allows the maximum amount of oxygenated blood to return to the brain as rapidly as possible after the blood has been displaced by the contrast agent. Second, it improves the arterial definition of the angiogram in that non-opacified blood provides a bolus effect aiding in the rapid delivery of the contrast agent to the posterior fossa.

*E.R. Squibb.
†Mallinckrodt Chemical Works.

Table 2-3
Dosage Schedule for Vertebral Angiography

Age (years)	Renografin 60® (cc)
0–1	2
2–3	3
4–6	4
7–10	5
11 and over	6

Subclavian Angiography

If selective vertebral artery catheterization cannot be performed because of atherosclerosis or excessive tortuosity of the subclavian artery, opacification of the posterior fossa can still be obtained by a flush injection into the subclavian artery. A large bore catheter with sideholes as well as endholes* is substituted and placed in the subclavian artery with its tip opposite the origin of the vertebral artery. Between 30 and 40 cc of Renografin 60 at a flow rate of 20 cc/second is adequate to obtain good visualization of the posterior fossa vessels.

Brachial Angiography

Brachial angiography is an alternate method of obtaining posterior fossa angiography when selective vertebral catheterization is contraindicated. The vertebral artery is opacified by the retrograde injection of contrast material under high pressure into the brachial artery. The brachial artery is punctured using a 16-gauge thin-wall Seldinger needle, with the cannula left in place. To obtain sufficient reflux of the contrast agent up the subclavian artery to the origin of the vertebral, 40 cc of Renografin 60 at a flow rate of 25 cc/second is generally adequate. Since it takes approximately one second for the contrast agent to flow from the injection site to the origin of the vertebral artery, appropriate allowances must be made in the programming sequence. An injection on the left side will opacify only the left vertebral artery (if the artery does not originate from the aorta). On the right side (except when the right carotid artery originates directly from the aortic arch), usually both the right vertebral and right carotid arteries will be opacified. Rarely, the right vertebral artery originates directly from the aorta in which case right brachial angiography will fail to opacify the right vertebral artery.

*7FR Polyethylene, I.D., 0.066 inch; O.D., 0.095 inch; Becton-Dickinson Company, New Jersey.

COMPLICATIONS

In a series of 5000 patients, Meaney found that inexperienced angiographers had an incidence rate of complications from two-and-a-half to three-and-a-half times greater than experienced angiographers.[2] This suggests that technical problems and protracted procedures are two major factors in the occurrence of complications. Lack of a trained team of nurses and technicians in the radiology suite and of nurses in the ward to take care of the patient during the initial 24 hours after an angiogram may contribute to the occurrence of complications.

Complications of vertebral angiography may be due either to local causes at the puncture site, or to catheter manipulations. Allergic complications secondary to reaction of the patient to the contrast agent may also occur, but these have, in recent years, become less frequent due to the use of less-toxic contrast agents.

Local Causes[2]

The most common local complications are bleeding and thromboembolism. Bleeding may occur either from multiple or eccentric needle punctures of the vessel and, when catheters are used, from multiple catheter changes. Poorly tapered catheters and excessive force when introducing the catheter into the artery may also result in hematoma formation. Generally, when a hematoma occurs during the procedure, several minutes of pressure applied manually or with a sandbag should control the bleeding. On occasions, the only method of adequate control is withdrawal of the catheter. It is possible for acute bleeding to occur minutes or hours after the catheter withdrawal. This is usually precipitated by excessive limb movements when the patient is returned to the ward.

Thrombosis with ischemia of the lower leg occurs much less frequently than bleeding. Utilizing oscillometric methods, Siegelman and associates reported 2.3 percent incidence of thromboembolism following femoral catheterization.[3] Almost all of their complications, however, were found in patients catheterized with catheters of size 5.6F (outside diameter 2.2 mm) or larger. There appears to be a direct relationship between the size of the catheter and the incidence of thromboembolism. Thrombosis in younger patients appears to be related to arterial spasm, which if severe can mimic thrombosis. The brachial artery particularly is prone to spasm. Prolonged procedures also have a higher complication rate of local thrombosis.[3,4] Recent reports have demonstrated the accumulation of thrombi on the outside of the catheter.[4] Investigators are now researching the possibility of applying a nonthrombogenic coating to the catheter which should reduce this risk.[5-7]

Arteriovenous fistulae, pseudoaneurysm formation, local infection, and thrombophlebitis may all occur following femoral puncture, but these are relatively rare complications.

Brachial plexus paralysis has been described as a major complication of the axillary approach but this can be avoided by meticulous technique and postangiographic care.[8]

Manipulative Causes[2]

Emboli secondary to catheter manipulation form one of the major sources of angiographic complications. The emboli may be dislodged from atherosclerotic lesions in the aorta or by excessive injection pressures. In the older age group, especially in patients with atherosclerotic vascular disease, emboli dislodged from the carotid or subclavian artery can lodge in the anterior or posterior circulation. In some hospitals, heparinization of the patient is carried out prior to angiography to prevent the formation of thrombi with subsequent embolization.[9] Thrombi are particularly likely to occur within the sideholes of sidehole catheters. Forcible injection can then dislodge the thrombi. Gas embolization from air entering the catheter system through loose-fitting connections can also occur.

Selective catheterization is extremely dangerous if the lumen of the vertebral artery is blocked by the catheter. Accordingly, the subclavian artery must be visualized under fluoroscopy so that a decision can be made as to whether or not the vertebral artery is sufficiently large to accept the catheter. Diminution in blood flow through the vertebral artery can transiently or permanently impair cervical spinal cord or brainstem function.

Catheter manipulations may also cause intimal dissection of the artery. This rarely involves the cerebral vessels, but dissection of the aorta can occur, especially with rigid catheters. In the author's experience, this has never occurred with the soft Hanafee catheter used for selective vertebral angiography. It is possible, however, for it to occur with vigorous manipulations of a guide wire. The hazard of broken guide wires has largely been eliminated with the development of internal safety wires bonded to the distal and proximal ends of the guide wire.

Subintimal injections and hematomas are the most common type of complication found after direct vertebral puncture techniques. Rarely, arteriovenous fistulae between the vertebral artery and the paravertebral venous plexus may result.[10,11]

The neurological deficits that occur following vertebral angiography are due either to compromise of the cerebral blood flow to the posterior circulation, or toxic effects of the contrast agent on the central nervous system. Temporary cortical blindness is reported to occur in about 1 percent of patients undergoing catheter vertebral angiography with methyl glucamine compounds.[12,13] More permanent complications that have been reported include transverse myelitis, paraplegia, basilar artery thrombosis, and hemiparesis.[2,14,15]

RADIOGRAPHIC TECHNIQUE

When possible, biplane simultaneous exposures of the frontal and lateral projections should be obtained so that the maximum information is obtained from a single injection. The lateral beam is centered approximately 3 cm above the external auditory canal. The frontal view is obtained as a semiaxial (Towne) projection, with the central ray angled 25° craniocaudad to the cathomeatal line and centered approximately 8 cm above the nasion. A supplementary view often obtained is an anteroposterior (Caldwell) projection, with the central ray angled 25° caudocraniad to the canthomeatal line. The beam should be centered on the acanthion. This view is ideal both for enface visualization of the basilar artery and its branches and for the evaluation of tonsillar herniation.

Magnification, utilizing x-ray focal spots of 0.3 mm or less, is an invaluable aid in providing high-quality and finely detailed images of the posterior fossa vasculature.

SUBTRACTION

The density of the petrous and facial bones often obscures visualization of the vessels of the posterior fossa and negates the effect of attaining high-detail anatomic images by the use of magnification techniques and small focal spots. It is possible to obtain sufficient penetration by overexposure, but again the superimposition of bone prevents adequate visualization of small vessels. In 1934, Ziedses des Plantes investigated the problem and suggested that a separate image of the difference between two radiographs obtained under similar conditions could be produced by covering one radiograph with a diapositive print of the other.[16] This essentially represents the subtraction technique in which the radiograph of the bone is subtracted from the radiograph of the bone with vessels. It is apparent that any movement of the bone between the two radiographs will preclude subtraction. For this reason, the image of the bone should be obtained immediately before the injection of the contrast agent. Since the patient may move during the passage of contrast agent through the head, an image of the bone should also be obtained at the end of the film series for a venous phase subtraction.

In obtaining the subtraction image, it is possible to utilize a diapositive of the radiograph without contrast agent for superimposition over the radiograph with contrast agent, *or* to utilize a diapositive of the radiograph with contrast for superimposition over the radiograph without contrast agent. Either method will give an adequate subtraction result as long as the density range in the diapositive is as great as in the original. The diapositive is called the *subtraction mask*. Many different types of radiographic film can be used to make a subtraction mask. The methods and films used as described below have proved adequate in the author's hands.

First Order Subtraction

1. Original radiograph with contrast agent in vessels—**A** (Fig. 2-1).

2. Place **A** on glass front of a photographic box in which the light originates from a bank of 12 bulbs with a total wattage of 24 watts. A timer allows any time from 0.5 to 30 seconds to be selected. Cover **A** with a sheet of Kodak RP/SU X-OMat Subtraction Films,* emulsion side down, and expose for approximately 3 to 4 seconds—**B** (Fig. 2-2).

3. Original radiograph without contrast agent—**C** (Fig. 2-3).

4. Superimpose **B** and **C** so that perfect registration is obtained. Tape the two films together.

5. Place combination **B** and **C** on glass front of photographic box, and cover with a sheet of Kodak RP/SU X-Omat Subtraction Film,* emulsion side down. Expose for approximately 3 to 4 seconds—**D** (Fig. 2-4).

6. Place **D** on the glass front, and cover with a sheet of DuPont Cronex Subtraction Film.† Expose for approximately 3 to 4 seconds—**E** (Fig. 2-5).

All films are processed in a 90-second X-OMat Processor.‡

It is difficult to obtain a complete cancellation of the bone with the method just outlined, since the density range of the subtraction mask is slightly less than that of the original. To increase the cancellation of the bone, two masks are prepared. The method is called second order subtraction.

*Kodak RP/SU X-OMat Subtraction Film.
†DuPont Cronex Subtraction Film.
‡Kodak M6 Processor.

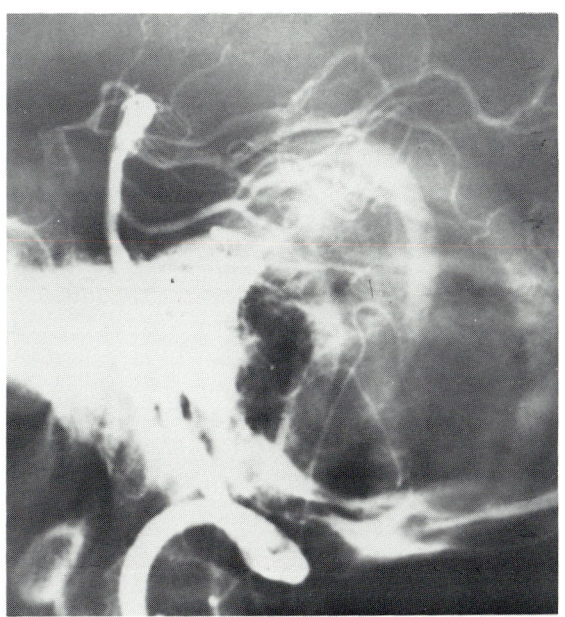

Fig. 2-1. First Order Subtraction. Original film with contrast agent.

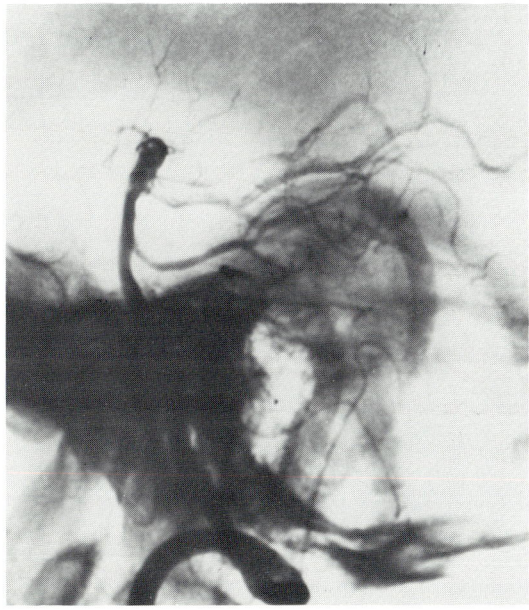

Fig. 2-2. First order subtraction. Original film reversed.

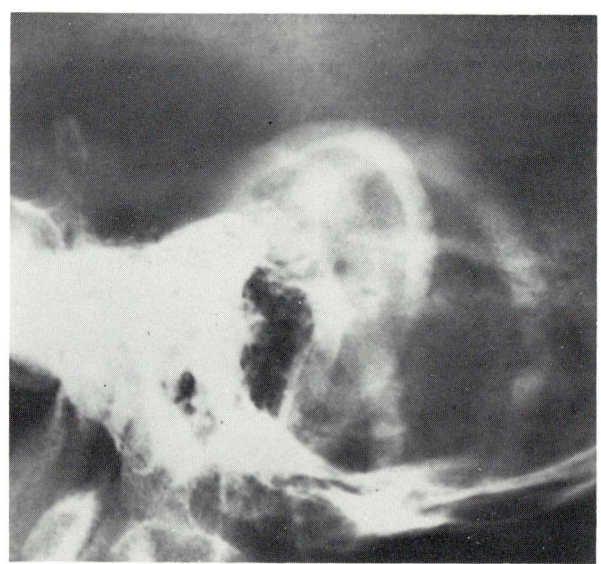

Fig. 2-3. First order subtraction. Original film without contrast agent.

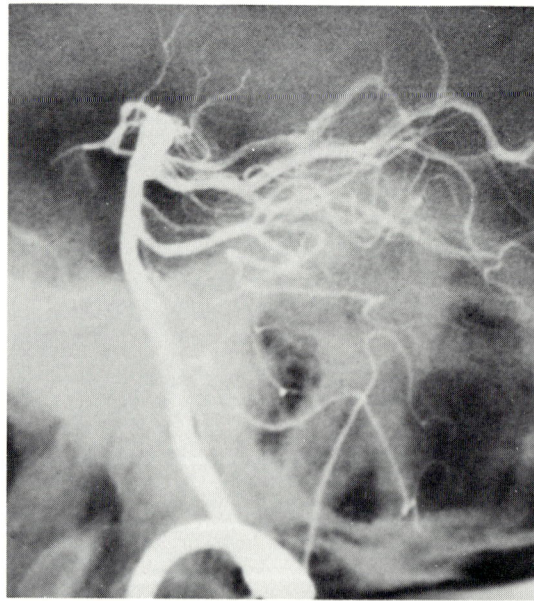

Fig. 2-4. First order subtraction. Result of superimposing Figs. 2-2 and 2-3.

Techniques of Vertebral Angiography

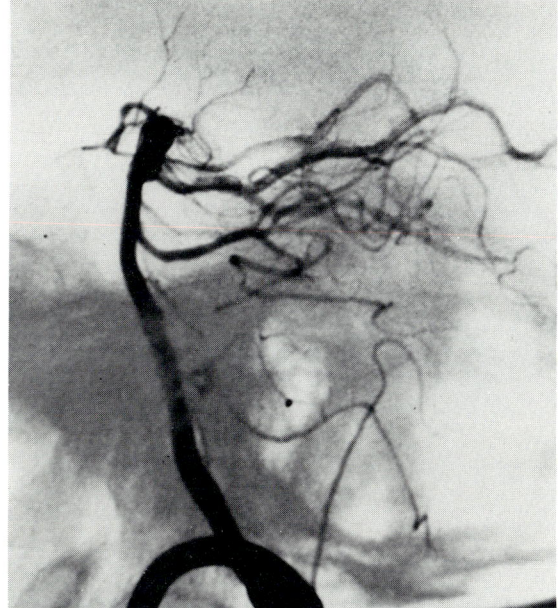

Fig. 2-5. First order subtraction. Reversal of Fig. 2-4.

Second Order Subtraction

1. Original radiograph without contrast agent in vessels—**A** (Fig. 2-6).

2. Place **A** on glass front, and superimpose Kodak RP/SU X-OMat Subtraction Film, emulsion side down. Expose for approximately 3 to 4 seconds—**B** (Fig. 2-7).

3. Superimpose **A** and **B** with perfect registration. Tape the two films together. Place combination on glass front, and superimpose Kodak RP/SU X-OMat Subtraction Film. Expose for approximately 3 to 4 seconds to obtain a second mask—**C** (Fig. 2-8).

4. Original radiograph with contrast agent—**D** (Fig. 2-9).

5. Superimpose **B** and **C** and **D**. Tape together. If combination is dark, place **B** and **C** and **D** on glass front, and cover with a sheet of Kodak RP/SU X-OMat Subtraction Film. Expose for approximately 7 to 9 seconds. If

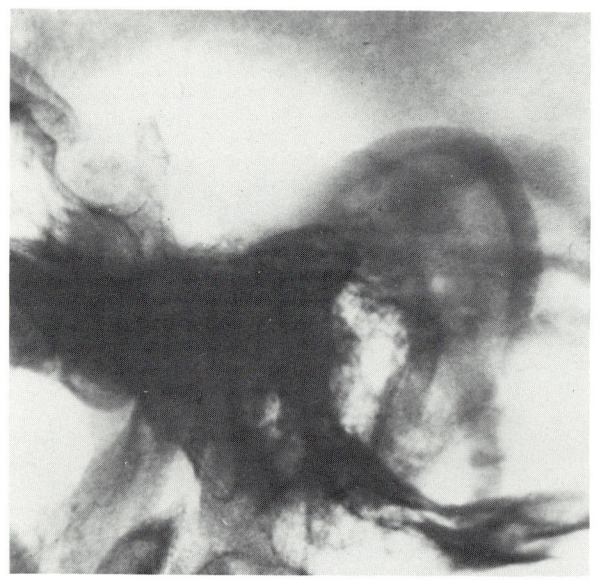

Fig. 2-6. Second order subtraction. Original film without contrast agent.

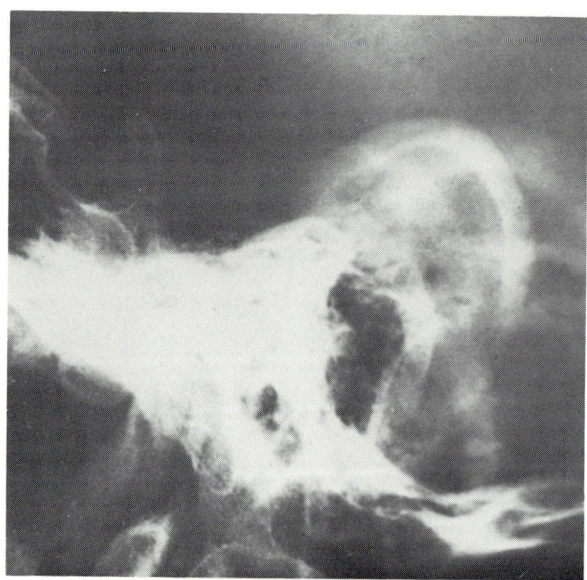

Fig. 2-7. Second order subtraction. Original film reversed.

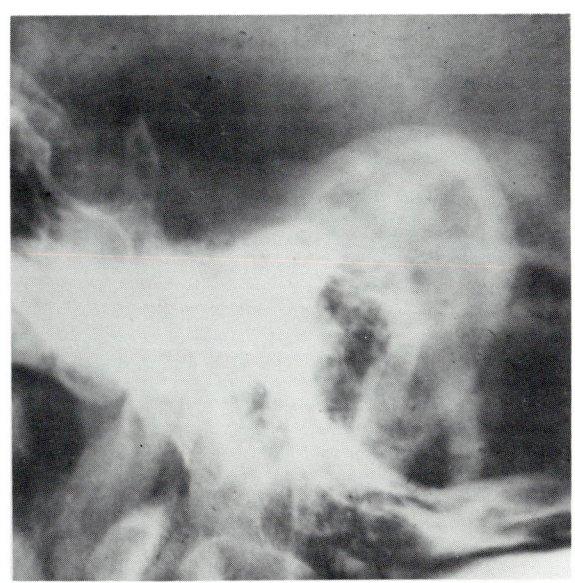

Fig. 2-8. Second order subtraction. Result of superimposing Figs. 2-6 and 2-7.

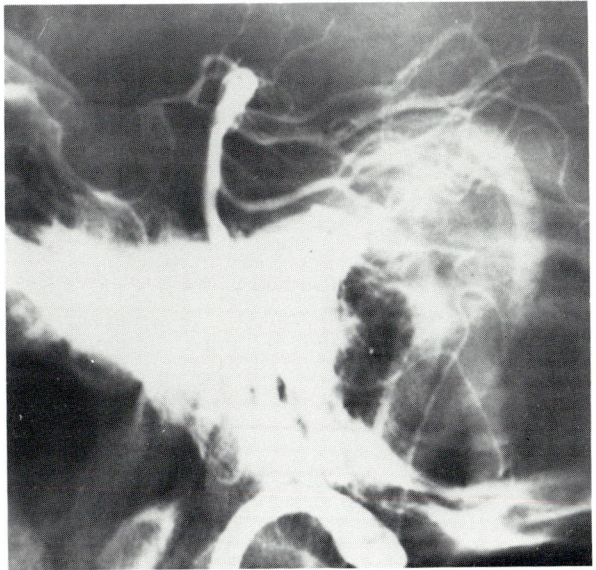

Fig. 2-9 Second order subtraction. Original film with contrast agent.

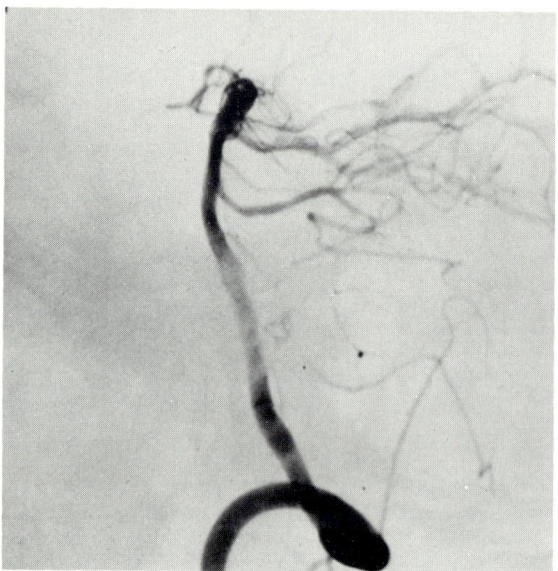

Fig. 2-10. Second order subtraction. Result of superimposing Figs. 2-7, 2-8, and 2-9.

initial combination is light, cover with a sheet of DuPont Cronex Subtraction 90-second film, and expose for 16 seconds—**E** (Fig. 2-10).

All films are processed in a 90-second X-OMat Processor.

ANGIOTOMOGRAPHY

Angiotomography is a technique for obtaining sharp images of the blood vessels in a selected plane while adjacent planes are blurred. Its value in posterior fossa angiography is mainly to define midline vessels such as the precentral cerebellar vein and anterior ponto-mesencephalic vein without the interference of adjacent hemispheric vessels. Angiotomography can be obtained by shaking the patient's head from side to side continuously during a relatively long lateral film exposure. A mechanical device is also commercially available in the form of a head cradle which provides the side-to-side rotation of the head about the cervical axis.* Films at approximately one-second intervals can be obtained from the arterial through to the venous phase of the angiogram with the Angiotome.

*Newton Angiotome, N&H Instruments, Inc., Carrollton, Texas.

REFERENCES

1. Heinz E R: Neuroradiologic special procedures, in Meaney T F, Lalli A F, Alfidi R J (eds): Complications and Legal Implications of Radiologic Special Procedures. St. Louis, Mosby, 1973
2. Meaney T F: Percutaneous femoral angiography, in Meaney T F, Lalli A F, Alfidi R J (eds): Complications and Legal Implications of Radiologic Special Procedures. St. Louis, Mosby, 1973
3. Siegelman S S, Caplan L H, Annes G P: Complications of catheter angiography: Study with oscillometry and "pullout" angiograms. Radiology 91:251, 1968
4. Formanek G, Frech R S, Amplatz K: Arterial thrombus formation during clinical percutaneous catheterization. Circulation 41:833, 1970
5. Amplatz K: A simple non-thrombogenic coating. Invest Radiol 6:280, 1971
6. Glancy J J, Fishbone G, Heinz E R: Nonthrombogenic arterial catheters. Am J Roentgenol 108:716, 1970
7. Jacobson B, Schlossman D: Thrombogenic properties of heparinised vascular catheters. Acta Radiol [Diagn] (Stockh) 14:569, 1973
8. Molnar W, Paul D J: Complications of axillary arteriotomies. An analysis of 1,762 consecutive studies. Radiology 104:269, 1972
9. Wallace S, Medellin H, de Jongh D, Gianturco C: Systemic heparinization for angiography. Am J Roentgenol 116:204, 1972
10. Lester J: Arteriovenous fistula after percutaneous vertebral angiography. Acta Radiol [Diagn] (Stockh) 5:337, 1966
11. Newton T H, Darroch J: Vertebral arteriovenous fistula complicating vertebral angiography. Acta Radiol [Diagn] (Stockh) 5:428, 1966
12. Wishart D L: Complications in vertebral angiography as compared to non-vertebral cerebral angiography in 447 studies. Am J Roentgenol 113:527, 1971
13. Horwitz N H, Wener L: Temporary cortical blindness following angiography. J Neurosurg 40:583, 1974
14. Howieson J, Megison L C, Jr: Complications of vertebral artery catheterization. Radiology 91:1108, 1968
15. Takahashi M, Kawanami H: Complications of catheter angiography: An analysis of 500 examinations. Acta Radiol [Diagn] (Stockh) 13:248, 1972
16. Des Plantes Z B G: Een methode om bepaalde onderdeelen van het röntgenologisch te onderzoeken voorwerp afzonderlijk in beeld te brengen. Ned Tijdschr Geneeskd 78:762, 1934

Bennett M. Stein

3
Clinical and Pathological Aspects of Posterior Fossa Tumors

SYNDROMES

Neurological syndromes produced by posterior fossa tumors are dependent on two major factors: (1) the destruction or compression of posterior structures by tumor; (2) obstruction of cerebrospinal fluid (CSF) leading to hydrocephalus due to a block of the sylvian aqueduct, fourth ventricle, or cisterns.[1-4]

In addition to these two major influences on the symptomatology is the importance of the rapidity of growth of the neoplastic process. Tumors that grow slowly may produce very few neurological signs since the parenchymal tissue adapts as it is slowly displaced by the expanding neoplasm. Conversely, neoplasms that grow rapidly tend to destroy tissue and produce a more overt neurological syndrome related to the structures involved.

Regional Involvement

CEREBELLUM

Tumors involving the cerebellar hemispheres produce a syndrome of limb ataxia.[2] This is manifested by incoordination of arm, hand, and finger movements, as well as a subordinate involvement of the less-skilled lower extremity. Defects are easily brought out by observing the patient's writing and other activities requiring precise coordination. Involvement of the cerebellar vermis produces a different picture of incoordination which is primarily confined to the trunk and to gait. The patient is unable to walk in a tandem fashion and, when standing or sitting, has difficulty in maintaining his postural equilibrium. In severe cases, the patient will reel from side to side so that he is unable to ambulate or stand.

FOURTH VENTRICLE

Tumors involving the fourth ventricle almost always compress or invade the floor of this structure.[4,5] Located in this region are many of the vital cranial nerve nuclei associated with eye, facial, and bulbar movements; the latter being related to speech, swallowing, and respiratory mechanisms. Therefore, such tumors may produce progressively severe vomiting early in their course and may in the late stages produce incapacitating bulbar symptomatology. Because of their strategic locations, tumors in this region are prone to produce obstruction of the CSF pathways and thereby a progressive rise in the intracranial pressure associated with hydrocephalus.

BRAINSTEM

Similar to those neoplasms involving the floor of the fourth ventricle are neoplasms which infiltrate the brainstem, such as the low-grade astrocytoma. They produce a plethora of cranial nerve findings as well as ataxia and paresis due to the interruption of cerebellar and corticospinal pathways.[4] Unlike tumors primarily within the fourth ventricle, however, tumors of the brainstem rarely produce obstruction; therefore, papilledema and hydrocephalus are usually not part of their clinical picture.

CEREBELLOPONTINE ANGLE

This region is a frequent location for acoustic neurinomas and, to a lesser extent, meningiomas. In this area lies a complex of cranial nerves subserving auditory, vestibular, facial motor, and facial sensory functions.[6] The acoustic tumor, which is the best example of a tumor in this region, produces deafness early, since it arises from the vestibular portion and compresses the auditory component of the eighth cranial nerve.[7] Subtle sensory and motor changes on the same side of the face are common. When these tumors grow to a large size, they involve the cerebellar connections in the cerebellum as well as in the brainstem and produce ataxia on the same side. Only late in their growth do these tumors both affect the bulbar cranial nerves and produce papilledema. Arterial involvement by these tumors may lead to indirect damage to the cochlear end organ as well as lateral portions of the pontine tegmentum.

PINEAL REGION

Neoplasms arising in this region, because of their proximity to the tectal region of the midbrain, produce a variety of cranial nerve defects primarily affecting the extraocular movements.[8] Typical of the syndrome is paralysis of upward gaze (Parinaud's syndrome). Unequal pupils with impaired reaction and convergence of the eyes have also been described. In addition, isolated defects of third and fourth nerve function may also be encountered. Because of the proximity of these neoplasms to the aqueduct, obstruction to CSF with hydrocephalus and evidence of intracranial hypertension are common. Continued growth of these neoplasms leads to ataxia and in some patients to precocious puberty and diabetes insipidus.

General Involvement

Blockage of the CSF pathways either in the aqueduct, fourth ventricle, or basal cisterns produces a syndrome of raised intracranial pressure. This is characterized by headache, which is most pronounced when the patient is straining or bending over. The headache tends to be persistent and is commonly noted in the morning. Vomiting is frequent. With either acute hydrocephalus or the latter stage of a chronic hydrocephalus, lethargy, confusion, or other supratentorial manifestations of the hydrocephalus may obscure the diagnosis of a posterior fossa tumor. Papilledema is common even without a fully developed syndrome of raised intracranial pressure and, therefore, can develop to a severe degree before the patient seeks medical attention. This may lead to immediate or delayed visual loss that is irreversible. Consequently, it is important to uncover the etiology of the raised intracranial pressure early in the course of posterior fossa neoplasms. Another frequent, but false, localizing sign related to raised intracranial pressure is the presence of a sixth nerve palsy. Generally, it does not signify direct involvement of the nerve, but rather an indirect effect due to a general increase in intracranial pressure.

PATHOLOGY

The overall incidence of brain tumors in the United States is in the range of 12,000 to 15,000 cases per year.[9] This includes primary as well as metastatic brain tumors.

In children, posterior fossa tumors which are intrinsic are the rule. In adults, other than metastatic lesions, intrinsic tumors are less common than those in extra-axial locations such as the cerebellopontine angle acoustic neurinomas.[10,11]

In children as well as adults, the type of tumor has a significant bearing on the surgical approach as well as what may be accomplished at surgery and thereby the prognosis.

Childhood Tumors

A characteristic feature of posterior fossa neoplasms is the well-known variation between type and location of tumors in children as compared with adults. In children, posterior fossa neoplasms comprise about 50 percent of all intracranial tumors, which rank third to those neoplasms that involve the lymphatic and renal systems.[10,11] In adults, while only 25 percent of central nervous tumors are located in the posterior fossa, the ratio of central nervous system tumors to systemic tumors is smaller. As the location of these tumors relates to the symptomatology, so the location of the tumor often relates to the histological nature of the tumor.

CEREBELLAR HEMISPHERE

Astrocytoma. In children, the cerebellar hemisphere is a common site for the cystic astrocytoma.[1,3,10] These tumors, growing insidiously and producing little in the way of symptomatology, are among the most benign of central nervous system tumors. Because of their slow growth, they often avoid clinical recognition and can attain enormous size before being diagnosed. The majority of these tumors are characterized by a large cyst containing highly proteinaceous fluid and a solid nodule located eccentrically in the mass. This has been referred to as a mural nodule and is discrete with a large portion of its surface presenting within the cystic cavity. The tumor nodule that is moderately vascular tends to present laterally in the cerebellar hemisphere and receives its blood supply primarily from the cerebellar arteries, whereas the cyst extends toward the midline and displaces the vermis so it's in relation to the roof or to the lateral portion of the fourth ventricle. The cyst wall of the tumor consists of compressed cerebellar tissue with a gliotic reaction. In the process of compression of cerebellar tissue, the surrounding vessels also become compressed by the tumor. The mural nodule or solid part of the tumor is invariably confined to cerebellar tissue, and although it may invade the cerebellar peduncles, it almost always stops short of the brainstem.

In rare instances, especially in the solid low-grade astrocytoma of the cerebellum, the tumor may be exophytic, growing outside the confines of the cerebellum into the lateral recesses of the fourth ventricle or growing via the cerebellar peduncles to invade the brainstem. The tumor is treated best by total excision, which can be accomplished in most instances.

CEREBELLAR VERMIS

Medulloblastoma. The vermis is the characteristic location for the highly malignant medulloblastoma.[5,12] This tumor is characteristically seen in childhood. It is highly vascular, rarely cystic, and infiltrates the surrounding cerebellar tissue. This tumor generally encroaches upon or fills the fourth ventricle and its interstices and invades the walls of the fourth ventricle. Interestingly, the tumor rarely invades the floor of the fourth ventricle, although, by virtue of its bulk, it can severely compress the brainstem and obstruct the flow of CSF. The tumor may also protrude from the posterior portion of the fourth ventricle, fill the cisterna magna and, occasionally, extend into the upper cervical region. Generally, the fourth ventricle, aqueduct, and other portions of the ventricular system dilate rostral to the tumor. Not only is the tumor capsule vascular, but the interior of the tumor is traversed by numerous blood vessels. Although these tumors are quite symmetrical in their growth from the midline, in about 10 percent of cases, they may occur primarily within the cerebellar hemisphere, in which case a modest-sized cyst containing from 10 to 15 cc of yellow fluid may be present. This is contrary to the cystic astrocytoma which often contains a large amount of fluid. The medulloblastoma has a propensity for seeding throughout the CSF spaces. In rare instances, the metastatic deposits may be the first sign of the tumor.

FOURTH VENTRICLE

As noted, the medulloblastoma, because of its rapid growth characteristic, tends to extend into and fill the fourth ventricle. There are, however, posterior fossa neoplasms in children that arise directly from within the fourth ventricle. These include the following:

Ependymoma. This tumor of intermediate malignancy is less common than the preceding two, is invasive, and may also seed throughout the CSF pathways, although not as frequently as the medulloblastoma.[13] It is a moderately vascular tumor originating from the ependymal surface of the fourth ventricle and invading the surrounding cerebellar tissue. It often intimately involves the posterior inferior cerebellar artery from which it may receive a major portion of its blood supply. Similar to the medulloblastoma, it displaces the brainstem anteriorly, but unlike the medulloblastoma, it often invades the fourth ventricle floor.

Choroid Plexus Papilloma. An uncommon tumor, the choroid plexus papilloma is benign and generally circumscribed, although in some cases it may extend out of the fourth ventricle. It usually is not attached to the walls of the fourth ventricle except in the region of the choroid plexus. It is highly vascular and receives its blood supply from those arteries which supply the choroid plexus. The tumor is slow growing and characteristically associated with an elevated CSF protein. Because of its moderately small size and insidious growth, symptoms may be nonexistent or minimal until obstruction of the fourth ventricle has occurred. In early stages, it may irritate the medullary vagal centers and produce vomiting and nystagmus due to involvement of the vestibular nuclei.

These tumors, lying in and around the fourth ventricle, usually receive their blood supply from the midline branches of the posterior inferior cerebellar artery. By comparison, the cystic cerebellar astrocytomas, lying within the hemisphere, can derive their blood supply from any or all of the three major cerebellar arteries.

BRAINSTEM

Astrocytoma. Generally, tumors that involve the brainstem are infiltrating and are of astrocytic origin.[5] Most of these tumors are low-grade astrocytomas; however, some may originate as or change into malignant types. They are generally slow growing and, because of their infiltrative nature, are slow to destroy brainstem function. Accordingly, tumors in this region may become quite large without severe neurological deficits. Because of the diffuse enlargement of the brainstem due to the tumor growth, the term pontine hypertrophy has been applied to the condition in the classic literature. Occasionally, the tumors may grow eccentrically, may even be exophytic, and thus produce large masses extending into the basal cisterns or the fourth ventricle. Especially noteworthy are the group of tumors that grow out of the brainstem via a small pedicle and come to lie almost totally in the cerebellopontine angle or fourth ventricle. These tumors have a different radiographic appearance than those diffusely infiltrating the brainstem. Such knowledge is invaluable to the neurosurgeon deliberating an exploration versus no exploration.

Brainstem tumors may originate in any region of the brainstem, from the mesencephalon to the medulla. Except for the rare instances of exophytic tumors, primarily cystic tumors, and intra-axial blood clots mimicking tumors, the vast majority of brainstem tumors are inoperable. Since brainstem tumors often respond poorly to surgery, it is important to recognize whether or not such a tumor is present and thereby avoid an unnecessary exploration.

Adult Tumors

Because of the different nature and location of posterior fossa tumors, these lesions prompt an entirely different set of considerations. In the adult, there is a high incidence of metastatic tumors that can implant throughout the cerebellum or the brainstem, although the usual site for these metastatic lesions is the cerebrum. They can also be multiple. With the exclusion of this tumor group, for practical purposes, primary tumors are extra-axial in location except for the uncommon hemangioblastoma.

CEREBELLUM

Hemangioblastomas. These tumors are usually cystic, may obtain a large size, and, like the cystic astrocytomas, have a nodule of tumor in one portion of the cyst.[14,15] This nodule is highly vascular and may assume the appearance of a vascular malformation on an angiographic study. The cyst is often of greater proportion in size than the solid nodule. The cerebellar hemisphere is the usual location for these masses, and their association with polycythemia is recognized. The mass effect of these lesions may obstruct the aqueduct and produce hydrocephalus. These lesions are benign and are usually moderately easy to resect.

EXTRA-AXIAL MASSES

Acoustic Neurinomas. These benign fibrous type tumors originate from the vestibular portion of the eighth cranial nerve. Depending on their exact origin in the course of the nerve, they may involve the acoustic canal, acoustic meatus, cerebellopontine angle cistern, or the brainstem. Many of these tumors are now diagnosed by sophisticated audiological testing when they are relatively small, in the range of 5 mm to 1 cm.[6,16] The evaluation of these patients, both prior to surgery as well as intraoperatively, is critically dependent on information regarding the displacements of adjacent blood vessels and of the brainstem itself.[7,17] These tumors are benign and can be totally resected. Their intimate relationship to the brainstem, blood vessels (especially the anterior inferior cerebellar artery), and the cranial nerves, however, makes their removal one of the most difficult tasks for the neurosurgeon to face.[18]

Meningiomas. A frequent location of these benign fibrous type of tumors is along the posterior surface of the petrous bone. They often extend into the cerebellopontine angle and along the clivus.[19] The tumors may also be located at the anterolateral margin of the foramen magnum. These tumors are not discrete, are ubiquitous in their growth, often spread throughout the posterior fossa, involve the cranial nerves as well as important arteries, and displace the brainstem. These features make total removal difficult.

SURGICAL CONSIDERATIONS

The posterior fossa, like no other region of the cranium, is tightly compacted with vital structures. Whereas supratentorial tumors, even those about the chiasm, may involve vital structures, none are as vital as the brainstem; injury to the brainstem will result in immediate or delayed death or, at the very least, in a vegetative state. Under these circumstances, room for surgical error is negligible. As a corollary, it is extremely difficult for a neurosurgeon to explore the posterior fossa in search of tumor pathology. The exposures tend to be limited. Even with large exposures, exploration of the contents including cerebellar hemispheres, vermis, brainstem, fourth ventricle, and the various cisterns is impractical. Therefore, it is extremly important in the preoperative evaluation that the precise location, size, and even nature of the tumor be defined. It is rare that this cannot be accomplished.

Even though thorough resection can do little for long-term survival in cases of highly malignant tumors such as medulloblastoma or ependymoma, surgery plays a role in unblocking the CSF passages and relieving acute hydrocephalus. Although it is useful to anticipate the histologic nature of tumors in the posterior fossa, it is not critical since these lesions all warrant exploration and resection of as much tissue as possible. Contrarily, brainstem tumors that can be verified preoperatively rarely require exploration which may be hazardous. An accurate assessment of the tumor's location and size obtained by radiological studies is more valuable than the knowledge of the histological nature of the lesion.

Small surgical exposures are predicted on an accurate assessment of the location of tumors. The routine exposures used are (1) midline suboccipital craniectomy, in which the large central area of the occipital bone is removed up to the transverse sinus, and the occipital sinus encountered in children divided; (2) the far lateral approach borders the sigmoid and lateral sinuses and is used for tumors of the cerebellopontine angle. Occasionally, it is important to know the patency and size of the venous sinuses involved in the event that these sinuses must be sacrificed; however, this is rarely necessary. In addition to these basic exposures, the rim of the foramen magnum is often removed, and, in the case of tonsillar herniation, the posterior arch of the first cervical vertebra is also removed. Because this requires additional exposure, it is important, if possible, to anticipate tonsillar herniation by the evaluation of preoperative radiographic studies. Upon opening the dura over the appropriate area, the tumor is usually readily visible.

Techniques of Evaluation

A fundamental question must be raised about the role of ventriculography or pneumoencephalography alone or in combination with angiography. The advantage of ventriculography is that it confirms the presence of neoplasm revealed by brain scan and angiography. It satisfactorily outlines the fourth ventricular component of the tumor by capping it with air or positive contrast media, which gives a clearer representation of the surface of the tumor and its contour.[20] Ventriculography also demonstrates the degree of obstruction to

CSF and the extent of hydrocephalus while permitting a decompression of the ventricular system. Pneumoencephalography permits an evaluation of the subarachnoid spaces and is particularly valuable in extra-axial tumors. The disadvantages of these studies are that they are time-consuming and may require general anesthesia. If followed by a definitive operation, they add inordinately to the time of the operative procedure. Sudden changes in intracranial pressure may be hazardous to the patient and, in addition, Pantopaque ventriculography can be irritating and produce an aseptic meningitis. Many neurosurgeons precede the definitive operative procedure on the tumor by a shunt in order to relieve the hydrocephalus and blunt the effects of raised intracranial pressure. This is generally more difficult to do following ventriculography than angiography. On balance, it appears that pneumography should be avoided if accurate information regarding the tumor size and location is obtainable from angiography and scan. Our personal experience is that, in most instances, information from angiography is sufficient to preclude ventriculography. This presupposes that the neuroradiologist uses all of his skills, including selective catheterization, various projections, magnification and subtraction techniques.

Special Circumstances

CEREBELLOPONTINE ANGLE

The common tumors occurring in this region are acoustic neurinomas and meningiomas. It is important for the surgeon to be able to appreciate the extent of the tumor from the degree of bone erosion, especially of the internal auditory meatus and canal.[6] The intimate involvement of the arterial tree by these tumors makes it mandatory that the course of the anterior inferior cerebellar artery be outlined.[18] This artery is often hidden from view during the initial surgical exposure; therefore, its radiographic position is of great assistance to the surgeon in his dissection. Furthermore, the position of this artery and adjacent veins helps to clarify the relation of the tumor to the brainstem.

FOURTH VENTRICLE

The exact position of tumors within the fourth ventricle, as to their symmetry, eccentricity, and the degree to which they fill the lateral recesses and cisterns, is extremely important in planning a surgical approach and tumor resection. Because of the close proximity of many tumors to the brainstem, it is important to know the rostral position of the fourth ventricle during surgical dissection. Major arteries encountered at the time of surgery are usually the posterior inferior cerebellar artery and its branches. Therefore, it is important to visualize their position on the preoperative angiogram, since they may be hidden by tumor during the initial exposure.

BRAINSTEM GLIOMAS

Although rare cases of benign cysts or blood clots mimicking tumors within the brainstem have been described, the vast majority of these lesions are infiltrative and not resectable. The clinical criteria for exploration include asymmetry of the clinical picture such as cranial nerve and cerebellar involvement on one side alone, the presence of papilledema, and a chronic history beginning primarily as a cerebellar disorder. The main question to ask the neuroradiologist is whether or not he is capable of unequivocally diagnosing these lesions as infiltrative brainstem gliomas without air-contrast studies.

PINEAL REGION TUMORS

The variety of tumor histology in this region, which includes a significant percentage of benign tumors, mandates surgical exploration of these lesions.[8] Since the approach differs, it is important to differentiate tumors that are primarily in the pineal region from those in the third ventricular or thalamic region, as well as from those of the anterior vermis. The vascular pattern within these different tumors may give some preoperative clue as to the histological nature of the lesion. At the present time, sufficient angiographic data correlated with histological specimens is not yet available to make a dogmatic statement regarding this feature.

Innovations

To relieve hydrocephalus, shunts are being performed with increasing frequency prior to definitive surgery on posterior fossa tumors that have obstructed the CSF flow. It would appear that the morbidity of patients treated by this approach is reduced. In such instances, it is valuable to know promptly as much about the tumor as can be obtained from radiological techniques. In addition to demonstrating ventricular size, angiography not only discloses the site and extent of the neoplasm but also, in many cases, defines the pathology.

The operating microscope is being used with increasing frequency in posterior fossa neoplasms. Since much of the dissection is carried out in a precise anatomical fashion with sharp dissection about the margins of the tumor and attention to vascular anatomy, it has been extremely useful to have an accurate assessment of the vascular anatomy in relationship to these neoplasms prior to surgical intervention.

In dealing with posterior fossa tumors where previously ventriculography and pneumoencephalography have been the stalwarts of the diagnostic procedures, angiography has taken the initiative. It simplifies the diagnostic evaluation, places less strain on the patient, and results in a more accurate appraisal of the pathology.

REFERENCES

1. Cushing H: Experiences with the cerebellar astrocytomas: A critical review of seventy-six cases. Surg Gynecol Obstet 52:129, 1931
2. Holmes G: Symptomology of cerebellar tumors; a study of for cases, in Sir Gordon Holmes: Selected Papers. London, MacMillan, 1956, pp 35–47
3. Matson DD: Cerebellar astrocytoma in childhood. Pediatrics 18:150, 1956
4. Wolf JK: The Classical Brainstem Syndromes. Springfield, Charles C. Thomas, 1971
5. Bray PF, Carter S, Taveras JM: Brainstem tumors in children. Neurology (Minneap) 8:1, 1958
6. Hanafee WN, Wilson GH: Pontocerebellar angle tumors, newer diagnostic methods. Arch Otolaryngol 92:236, 1970
7. Pool JL, Pava AA, Greenfield EC: Acoustic Nerve Tumors. Early Diagnosis and Treatment (ed 2). Springfield, Charles C. Thomas, 1969
8. Stein BM: The infratentorial supracerebellar approach to pineal lesions. J Neurosurg 35:197, 1971
9. Youmans JR (ed): Neurological Surgery. Philadelphia, Saunders, 1973, p 1320
10. Bailey P, Buchanan DN, Bucy PC: Intracranial Tumors of Infancy and Childhood. Chicago, University of Chicago Press, 1939
11. Matson DD: Neurosurgery of Infancy and Childhood (ed 2). Springfield, Charles C. Thomas, 1969
12. Crue BL, Jr: Medulloblastoma. Springfield, Charles C. Thomas, 1958
13. Kricheff II, Becker M, Schneck SA, Taveras JM: Intracranial ependymoma: A study of survival in 65 cases treated by surgery and irradiation. Am J Roentgenol 91:167, 1964
14. Green JR, Vaughan RJ: Blood vessel tumors and hematomas of the posterior fossa in adolescence. Angiology 23:474, 1972
15. Palmer JJ: Haemangioblastomas. Acta Neurochirurgica 27:125, 1972
16. Jerger J: Review of diagnostic audiometry. Ann Otol Rhinol Laryngol 77:1042, 1968
17. Mazzoni A, Hansen CC: Surgical anatomy of the arteries of the internal auditory canal. Arch Otolaryngol 91:128, 1970
18. Atkinson WJ: The anterior inferior cerebellar artery: its variations, pontine distribution, and significance in surgery of cerebello-pontine angle tumours. J Neurol Neurosurg Psychiatry 12:137, 1949
19. Castellano F, Ruggiero G: Meningiomas of the posterior fossa. Acta Radiol [Diag] (Suppl) (Stockh) 104:1, 1953
20. Hilal SK, Tookoian H, Wood EH: Displacement of the aqueduct of sylvius by posterior fossa tumors. Acta Radiol [Diagn] (Stockh) 9:167, 1969

4
Normal Angiographic Anatomy of Posterior Fossa
(Plates I and II*)

VERTEBRAL ARTERY

The vertebral artery normally arises as the first and largest branch of the subclavian artery.[1] It arises from the cranial surface of the convexity of the arch of the subclavian artery. (In older people with tortuosity of the subclavian artery, the point of origin becomes more medial and anterior. Catheterization of the artery is, accordingly, more difficult in the elderly.) The artery enters the transverse process of the sixth cervical vertebra and ascends through the foramina of the transverse processes to the foramen transversarium of the third cervical vertebra (Fig. 4-1). It then proceeds laterally to the foramen transversarium of the atlas. Emerging from this foramen, it swings directly posteriorly and then medially around the lateral surface of the superior articular process of the atlas to lie in a grove on the cranial surface of the posterior arch of the atlas. (According to Brain, the loop made by the vertebral artery around the atlas and the loop made by the carotid artery in its cavernous portion cause a damping effect on the blood pressure and aid in the regulation of cerebral blood flow.)[2] The vertebral artery penetrates the dura mater and arachnoid immediately below the skull and enters the cranial cavity through the foramen magnum. It then courses superiorly, anteriorly, and medially to unite with the contralateral vertebral artery at approximately the lower border of the pons to form the basilar artery (Fig. 4-2).[3]

The artery can be divided into four parts.[1]

*See color plates, page 33.

Plate I. Normal Inferior Cerebellar Anatomy (Chapter 4). On the frontal diagram *(left)*, note the origins of the posterior inferior cerebellar arteries (PICA) from the vertebral arteries and their relationships to the medulla and cerebellar hemispheres. The red dashes indicate the arteries as seen through the cerebellum on its undersurface. The inferior vermian veins are also shown.

On the lateral diagram *(right)*, the following vessels are shown: vertebral artery, basilar artery, posterior inferior cerebellar artery and branches, superior cerebellar artery, inferior vermian and superior vermian veins, ponto-mesencephalic vein, precentral cerebellar vein, great vein of Galen, straight sinus, and torcula.

Plate II. Normal Superior Cerebellar Anatomy (Chapter 4). On the frontal diagram *(left)*, note the relationship of the superior cerebellar arteries and branches to the upper pons and superior hemispheric surfaces.

The lateral diagram *(right)* depicts the same vessels as shown in Plate I.

Plate III. Prepontine and Cerebellopontine Angle Tumors (Chapter 5). The upper two diagrams demonstrate the normal vascular anatomy. Note on the frontal diagram *(upper left)*, the relationships of the anterior inferior cerebellar artery and the petrosal vein to the anterior surfaces of the cerebellum.

In the lower left diagrams, the cerebellopontine angle tumors as they grow out of the internal auditory canals are shown displacing the anterior inferior cerebellar artery and the petrosal vein superiorly.

In the lower right diagram, note the posterior displacement of the basilar artery and ponto-mesencephalic vein by a prepontine tumor.

In the series of color plate diagrams, the cerebrospinal fluid pathways are yellow; the arteries, red; the veins, blue; the cerebellar hemispheres, dark gray; the pons and medulla, light gray; and the tumors, green.

The plates are diagrammatic and should be analyzed in conjunction with the relevant chapters.

Only major vessel displacements are indicated.

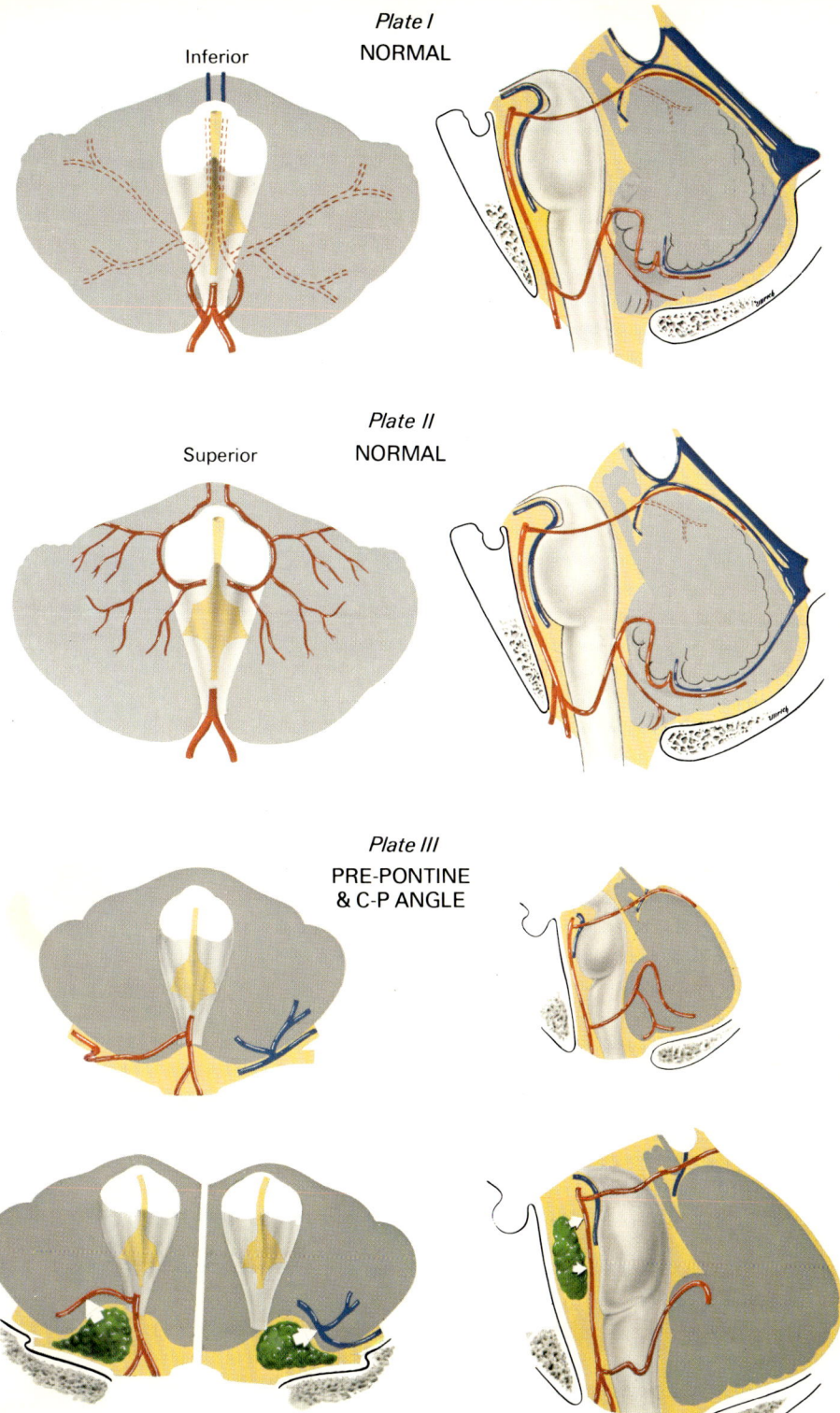

Plate IV
PONS & MIDBRAIN

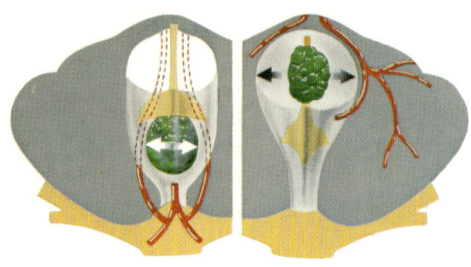
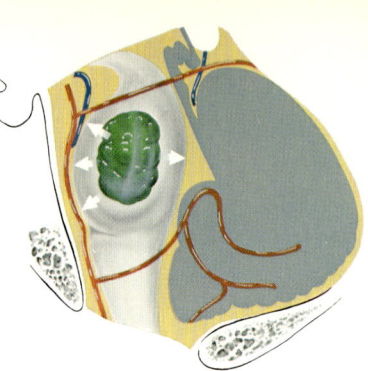

Plate V
FOURTH VENTRICLE

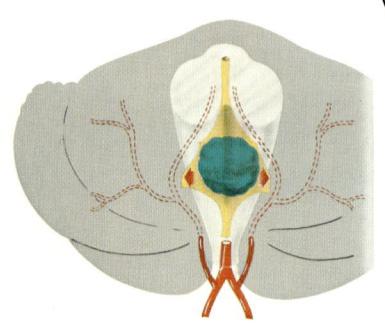
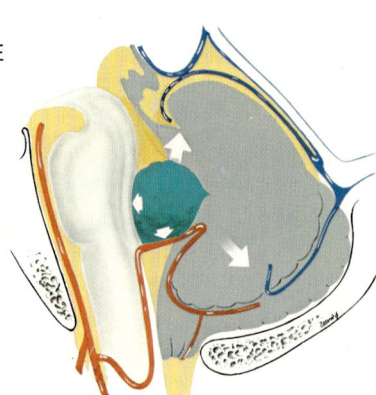

Plate VI
INFERIOR VERMIS & HEMISPHERE

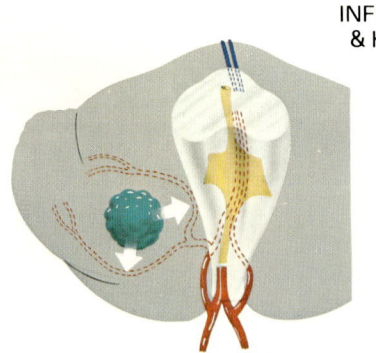
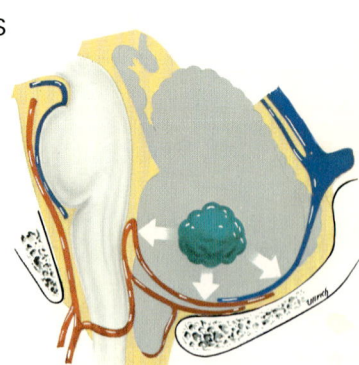

Plate VII
SUPERIOR VERMIS & HEMISPHERE

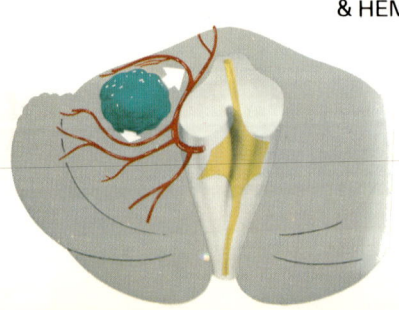
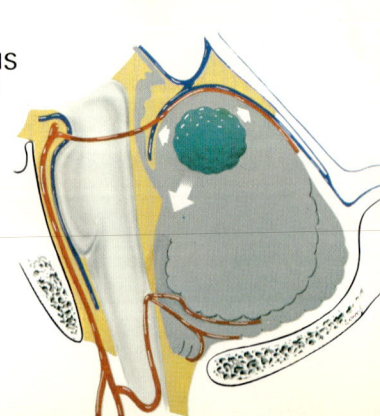

Normal Angiographic Anatomy of Posterior Fossa

Plate IV. Pontine and Mesencephalic Tumors (Chapter 6). The left diagrams demonstrate the effect of a medullary tumor on the posterior inferior cerebellar arteries and of a midbrain tumor on the superior cerebellar arteries. The effect on the posterior inferior cerebellar arteries is usually surprisingly minimal due to invasion of the adjacent cerebellar hemisphere by tumor (see Chapter 6, Fig. 6-13, p. 128).

In the right diagram, a midpontine tumor is shown displacing the basilar artery and ponto-mesencephalic vein anteriorly and the choroidal point of PICA and the precentral cerebellar vein posteriorly. With large tumors, there is also stretching of the medullary segments of PICA and of the perimesencephalic segments of the superior cerebellar artery.

Plate V. Fourth Ventricle Tumors (Chapter 7). The left diagram demonstrates separation of the supratonsillar and retrotonsillar segments of PICA.

The right diagram demonstrates stretching of the supratonsillar segment and posterior displacement of the retrotonsillar segment of PICA. It also demonstrates posterior displacement of the copular venous point and superior displacement of the precentral cerebellar vein. The basilar artery is displaced anteriorly. The ponto-mesencephalic vein (not shown) is also displaced anteriorly.

Plate VI. Inferior Vermian and Hemispheric Tumors (Chapter 8). The left diagram demonstrates the frontal view of an inferior hemispheric tumor as it displaces and stretches the posterior inferior cerebellar artery, its branches, and the inferior vermian veins.

The right diagram demonstrates the direct effect of an inferior vermian tumor displacing the choroidal point of the posterior inferior cerebellar artery anteriorly and its vermian branch inferiorly. Note the herniation of the tonsil and the tonsillohemispheric branch of PICA through the foramen magnum. The inferior vermian vein is displaced inferiorly and the basilar artery and ponto-mesencephalic vein anteriorly.

Plate VII. Superior Vermian and Hemispheric Tumors (Chapter 8). On the left diagram, a superior hemispheric tumor is seen displacing and stretching the hemispheric branches of the superior cerebellar artery.

On the right diagram, the tumor is seen displacing the superior vermian branch of the superior cerebellar artery superiorly and the precentral cerebellar vein anteriorly. The remote effect of the tumor is to displace the posterior inferior cerebellar artery inferiorly, the basilar artery anteriorly, and the ponto-mesencephalic vein anteriorly.

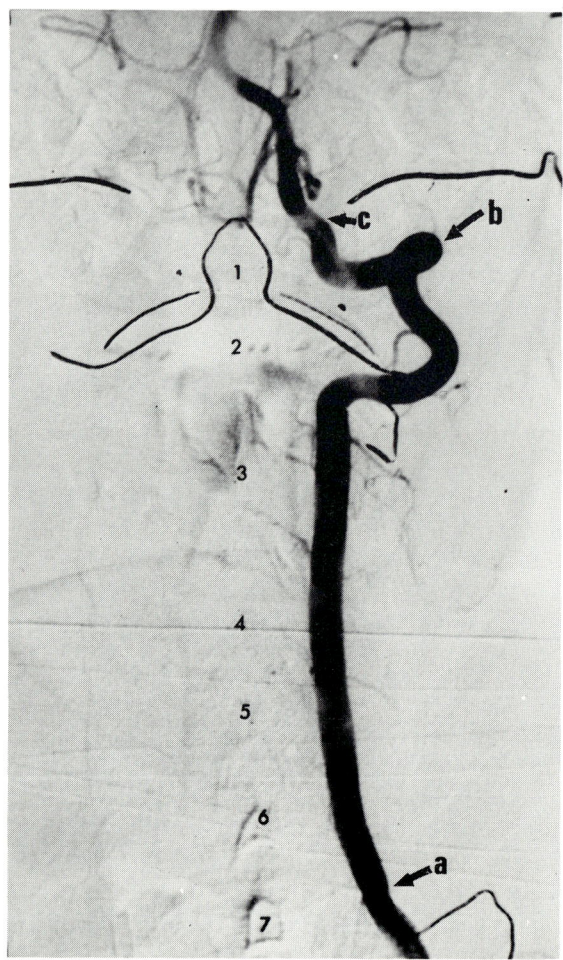

Fig. 4-1. Left vertebral angiogram, arterial phase, frontal projection. The left vertebral artery after originating from the subclavian artery courses through the foramina of C7 to C1. The first part is from its origin up to the foramen transversarium of C7 (a). The second part lies between a and b. Arrow b marks the point where the artery turns medially on top of the arch of the atlas. The third part is represented by the segment of the artery on top of the atlas (between b and c). The fourth part extends from the point of dural penetration (c) to the junction with the contralateral vertebral artery.

Normal Angiographic Anatomy of Posterior Fossa

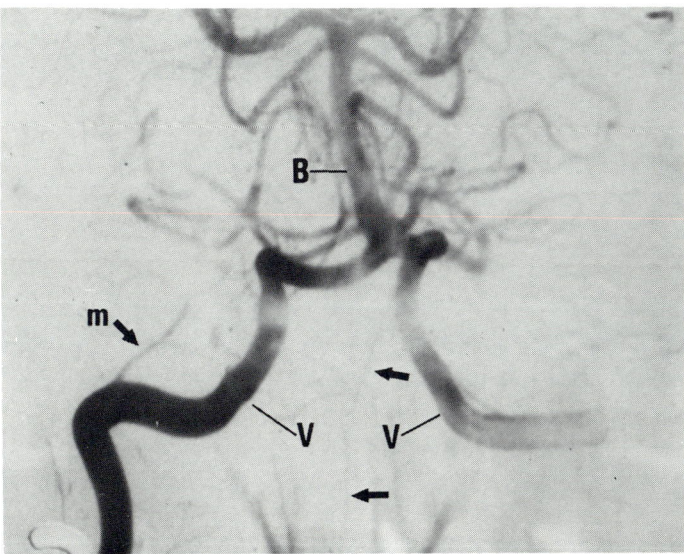

Fig. 4-2. Right vertebral angiogram, arterial phase, frontal projection: same case as Fig. 4-3. The two vertebral arteries (V) unite to form the basilar artery (B). The right vertebral (reader's left) is larger than the left. The anterior spinal artery (arrow) originates from the left vertebral artery and descends on the anterior surface of the spinal cord. A muscular branch (m) of the right vertebral artery supplies the occipital musculature.

1. From its origin to its entry into the foramen of the sixth cervical vertebra.
2. Through the transverse foramina of the sixth through the first cervical vertebrae.
3. From the foramen transversarium of C1 medially on the upper surface of the atlas to the point of dural penetration.
4. From the point of dural penetration to the union with the contralateral vertebral artery.

The second part is surrounded by branches from the inferior cervical sympathetic ganglion and by a plexus of veins originating from the internal vertebral venous plexus and small muscular veins.[1]

The sympathetic fibers accompany the vertebral and basilar arteries to the junction of the posterior cerebral and posterior communicating arteries. The fibers terminate at this point since the distal portion of the posterior cerebral artery is a continuation of the posterior communicating artery and, therefore, embryologically forms a part of the the internal carotid system. Thus, the posterior cerebral artery reflects its embryological origin by being supplied proximally by the vertebral plexus and distally by the carotid plexus.[4]

Branches

The branches may be divided into two sets—cervical and intracranial.[1]

Cervical Branches

The cervical branches can be subdivided into spinal and muscular branches.

Spinal Branches

Spinal branches enter the vertebral canal through the intervertebral foramina. These branches, in turn, divide into smaller branches supplying the cord and the vertebral bodies. The branches supplying the cord accompany the roots of the spinal nerves and reinforce the anterior and posterior spinal arteries. Often the upper cervical cord is supplied only by a single radicular artery accompanying the third cervical spinal nerve root. The branches supplying the vertebral bodies have cranial and caudal divisions forming anastomotic chains on the dorsal surface of the vertebral bodies and supply the underlying bone and periosteum.

Muscular Branches

Muscular branches usually originate from the vertebral artery as it curves around the articular process of the atlas and supply the deep muscles of the neck (Figs. 4-2, 4-3). They may anastomose with the occipital artery, the ascending pharyngeal artery, or the subclavian artery.[5-7] Muscular branches can also anastomose with the thyrocervical trunk, the costocervical trunk, or the transverse cervical artery.

Intracranial Branches

There are five main intracranial branches: meningeal, anterior spinal, posterior spinal, medullary, and posterior inferior cerebellar arteries.

Meningeal Arteries

The meningeal arteries originate from the fourth part of the vertebral artery and supply part of the dura of the posterior fossa (see p. NN).[1]

Anterior Spinal Artery

The anterior spinal artery is formed by the union of two main branches that originate from the medial surfaces of the fourth parts of the vertebral arteries. The two branches usually unite at the level of the foramen magnum corresponding to the level of the pyramidal decussation.[1,8] On occasions, the two branches may not unite and may continue caudally as separate trunks.[9] Only one branch continuing caudally as a single vessel can also occur.[3] As a common trunk, the artery descends along the ventral surface of the spinal cord and supplies the median-paramedian aspect of the medulla oblongata (Figs. 4-2, 4-3, 4-11). The anterior spinal artery was identified on lateral cervical films in 24 percent of brachial angiograms, 51 percent of direct puncture vertebral angiograms, and 94 percent of catheter vertebral angiograms.[9-11] The anterior spinal artery is seen more commonly on angiography then the posterior spinal artery.[12]

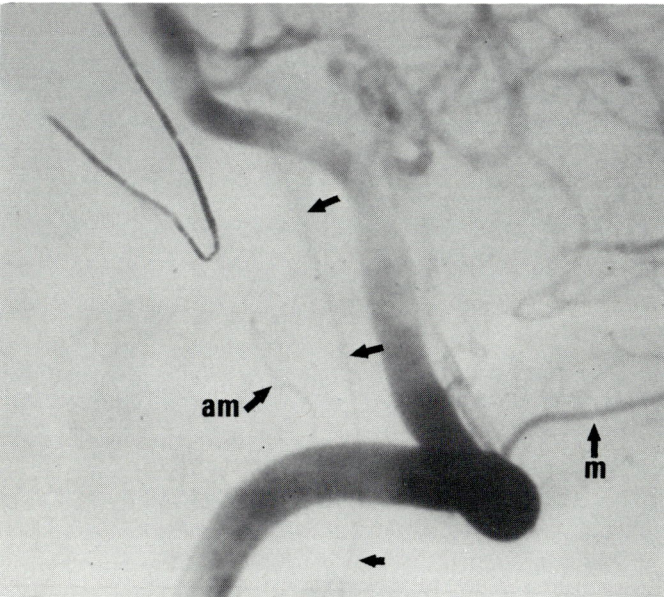

Fig. 4-3. Lateral projection. The anterior spinal artery (arrows) can be seen descending on the anterior surface of the spinal cord. The anterior meningeal artery (am) originates from the third portion of the vertebral artery and extends anterosuperiorly to supply the dura over the clivus. The muscular branch (m) of the vertebral artery is seen extending posteriorly.

Posterior Spinal Artery

The posterior spinal artery usually arises from the posterior medullary segment of the posterior inferior cerebellar artery, although it can arise directly from the fourth part of the vertebral artery.[1, 3, 13] It may receive a major branch from the opposite posterior inferior cerebellar artery, in which case the two branches unite behind the medulla to form a single trunk.[13] As the posterior spinal artery descends on the dorsal surface of the spinal cord, it receives a succession of spinal branches.[1] The percentage of visualization ranged between 4 percent and 38 percent of normal lateral angiograms in two different series.[9, 11]

Medullary Arteries

The medullary arteries are several minute vessels originating from the vertebral artery and its branches and are distributed to the medulla oblongata.[1] They have not been identified angiographically.

Posterior Inferior Cerebellar Artery

The posterior inferior cerebellar artery (PICA) is the largest branch and originates from the fourth part of the vertebral artery. After supplying the lateral and posterior medulla, it supplies the posterior inferior quadrant of the cerebellar hemisphere including the tonsil, the choroid plexus of the fourth ventricle, and inferior part of the vermis. The posterior inferior cerebellar artery has been described as passing between the rootlets of the hypoglossal nerve and then behind the rootlets of the glossopharyngeal and vagus nerves.[8] Between its point of origin and the vermian segment, however, the artery is subject to many variations, and the relationship of the artery to the lower cranial nerves varies considerably. The following description will be concerned with the usual course of the artery (Figs. 4-4 to 4-8). Variations will be described subsequently (see pp. 47–51).

After its origin from the vertebral artery, the PICA initially lies anterior to the medulla. This segment is known as the anterior medullary segment.[14] The artery then proceeds around the medulla, as the lateral medullary segment, describing a caudal loop convex inferiorly. The artery reaches the posterior margin of the medulla where it is called the posterior medullary segment. Greitz and Sjögren call the anterior and lateral medullary segments the cisternal part and the posterior medullary segment the medullary part.[15] The posterior medullary segment in the semiaxial projection is usually convex medially due to bulging of the anteromedial surface of the tonsil into the vallecula.[16] The

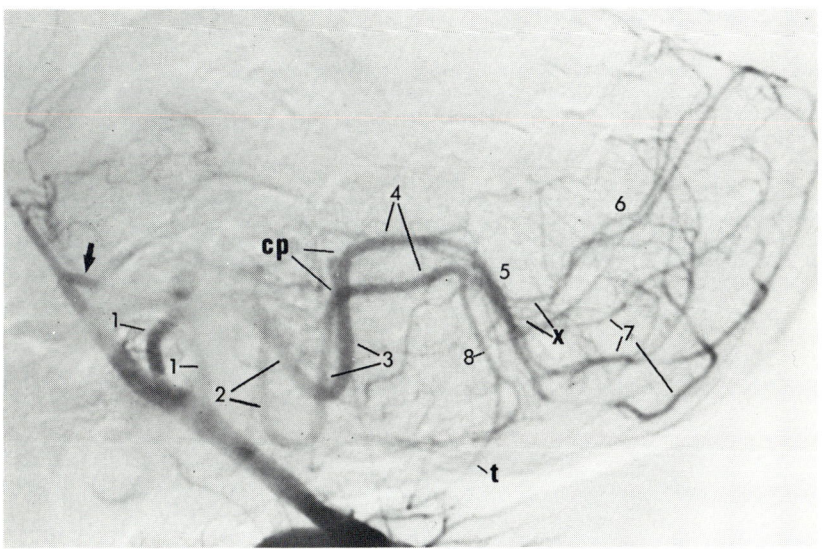

Fig. 4-4. Left vertebral angiogram, arterial phase, lateral projection: same case as Fig. 4-5. Both posterior inferior cerebellar arteries are seen originating from the vertebral arteries as anterior medullary segments (1), then extending lateral to the medulla as lateral medullary segments that make caudal loops convex inferiorly (2). The choroidal points (cp) of both posterior inferior cerebellar arteries are located at the junction of the ascending posterior medullary segments (3) and the supratonsillar segments (4). As the supratonsillar segment on the left is lower than that on the right, the choroidal points are at different heights and bear different relationships to the fastigium of the fourth ventricle. The retrotonsillar segments (5) are continuations of the supratonsillar segments and lie behind the tonsil. They then loop under the pyramidal lobe of the inferior vermis and continue as the inferior vermian branches (6). The most anteroinferior points on the pyramidal loops are called the copular points (x). The inferior hemispheric branches of the posterior inferior cerebellar artery (7), which run on the undersurface of the cerebellar hemisphere, arise from the retrotonsillar segments —which is unusual. They usually originate from the tonsillohemispheric branches (8) which are seen running posterior to the tonsil and subsequently on its undersurface (t). The hemispheric branches (7) project closer to the occipital bone than the inferior vermian branches (6) which are separated from the occipital lobe by the vermian cleft. The anterior cerebellar artery (arrow) is shown originating from the basilar artery which is occluded at the level of the superior cerebellar arteries.

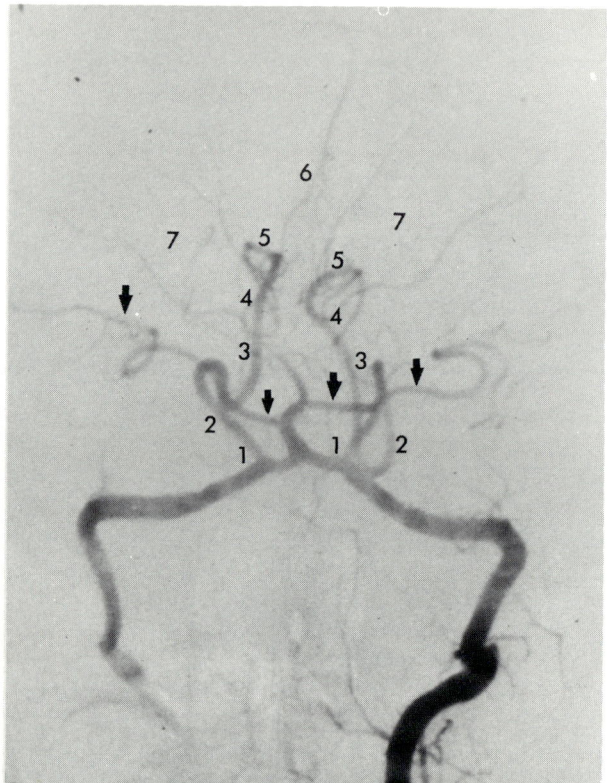

Fig. 4-5. Frontal projection. The occlusion of the basilar artery allows an unimpeded view of the posterior inferior cerebellar arteries and their branches. After originating from the vertebral arteries as the anterior medullary segments (1), the arteries loop inferiorly as the lateral medullary segments (2). Bulging of the tonsil into the vallecula causes the slight medial convexity of the posterior medullary segment (3) on the patient's right side (reader's left). On the patient's left side, the supratonsillar segment (4) is deviated medially by the tonsil. Hemispheric branches (7) fan out laterally. The anterior inferior cerebellar arteries (arrows) extend laterally into the cerebellopontine angle.

posterior medullary segment turns abruptly upward and ascends medial to the tonsil to its anterosuperior pole.

The PICA continues over the superior pole of the tonsil as the supratonsillar segment.[14] At this point, it forms a loop convex superiorly called the cranial loop or choroid arch.[15-17] Depending on whether the inferior medullary velum

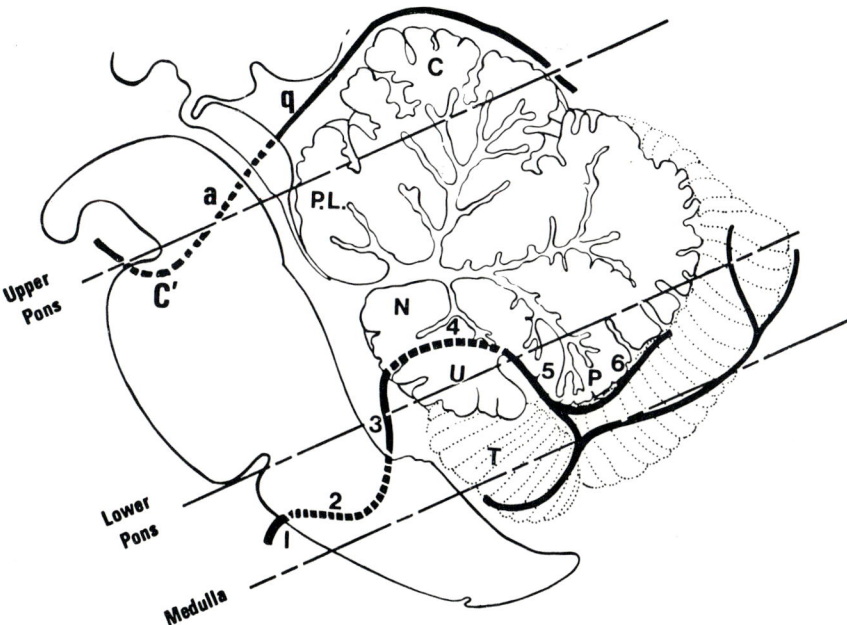

Fig. 4-6. Line diagram of a sagittal section of the pons and cerebellum. Note the relationship of the anterior medullary (1), lateral medullary (2), posterior medullary (3), supratonsillar (4), retrotonsillar (5), and inferior vermian (6) segments of the posterior inferior cerebellar artery to the medulla, nodulus (N), uvula (U), tonsil (T), and pyramis (P). The tonsillohemispheric branch is not numbered but is seen to originate from the retrotonsillar segment. The superior cerebellar artery is shown surrounding the upper pons with an initial downward loop called the crural-interpeduncular segment (C'). The ambient segment (a) surrounds the midbrain and then lies in the quadrigeminal cistern above the precentral lobule (P.L.). The segment within the cistern is called the quadrigeminal segment (q). Ascending over the culmen (C) the artery terminates in the midline as the superior vermian segment. Horizontal sections through the plane of medulla, lower pons, and upper pons are indicated and demonstrated in Figs. 4-20, 4-15, and 4-24 respectively.

is attached high or low with relation to the nodulus, the cranial loop will bear a variable relationship to the fastigium of the fourth ventricle.[17] Rarely does the cranial loop ascend as far superiorly as the fastigium. Usually, the cranial loop reaches up to the inferior medullary velum or lies 5 to 10 mm below it and sends small branches to supply the choroid plexus.[16] The junction of the posterior medullary segment and the supratonsillar segment is called the choroidal

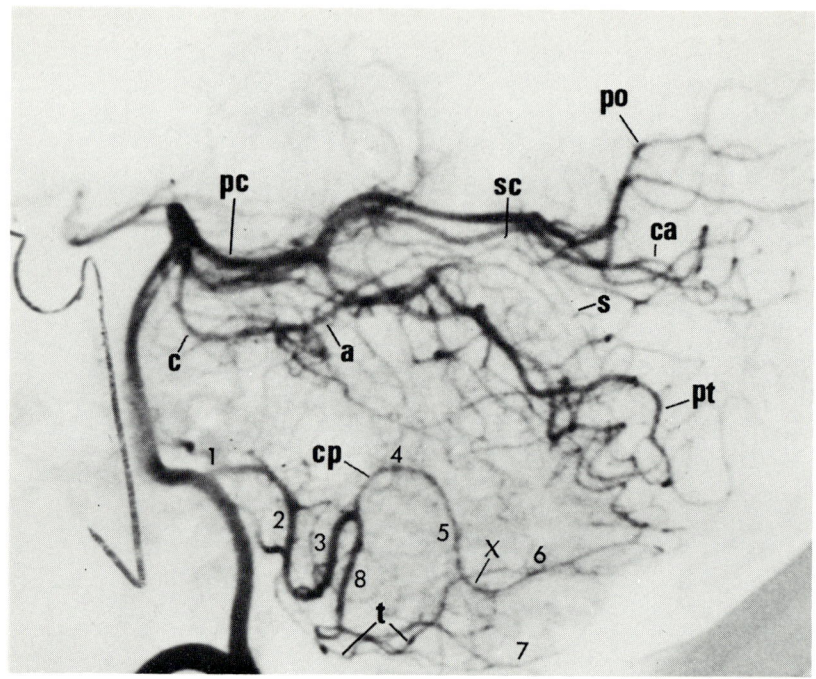

Fig. 4-7. Left vertebral angiogram, arterial phase, lateral projection: same case as Fig. 4-8. After originating from the vertebral artery as the anterior medullary segment (1), the lateral medullary segment (2) of the posterior inferior cerebellar artery dips downward alongside the medulla. Curving posteriorly, the artery lies adjacent to the posterior surface of the medulla as the posterior medullary segment (3). The choroidal point (cp) is at the junction of the posterior medullary and supratonsillar (4) segments of PICA. The tonsillohemispheric branch (8) originates from the posterior medullary segment and after supplying the tonsil with tonsillar branches (t) distributes hemispheric branches (7) on the undersurface of the cerebellar hemisphere. The retrotonsillar branch (5) of PICA lies behind the tonsil and terminates as the inferior vermian segment (6). Lying deep in the vermian cleft, the inferior vermian segment is separated from the occipital bone. The convex curvature at the junction of the retrotonsillar and inferior vermian segments constitutes the copular point (X).

The crural segment (c) of the superior cerebellar artery has an inferior convex curve. The ambient segment (a) is crossed by the posterior temporal branch (pt) of the posterior cerebral artery. The superior cerebellar artery continues onward and curves over the culmen of the cerebellum as the supraculminate segment (sc). The superior vermian branch (s) descends over the declive. The posterior cerebral artery (pc) has a convex curve parallel to that of the crural segment of the superior cerebellar artery. The parieto-occipital (po) and calcarine (ca) branches of the posterior cerebral artery originate from a common trunk (the internal occipital artery). The posterior temporal branch of the posterior cerebral artery is the most inferior branch of the posterior cerebral artery on the lateral projection. The slope of the tentorium dictates that the laterally situated posterior temporal branch should lie below the medially situated parieto-occipital branch.

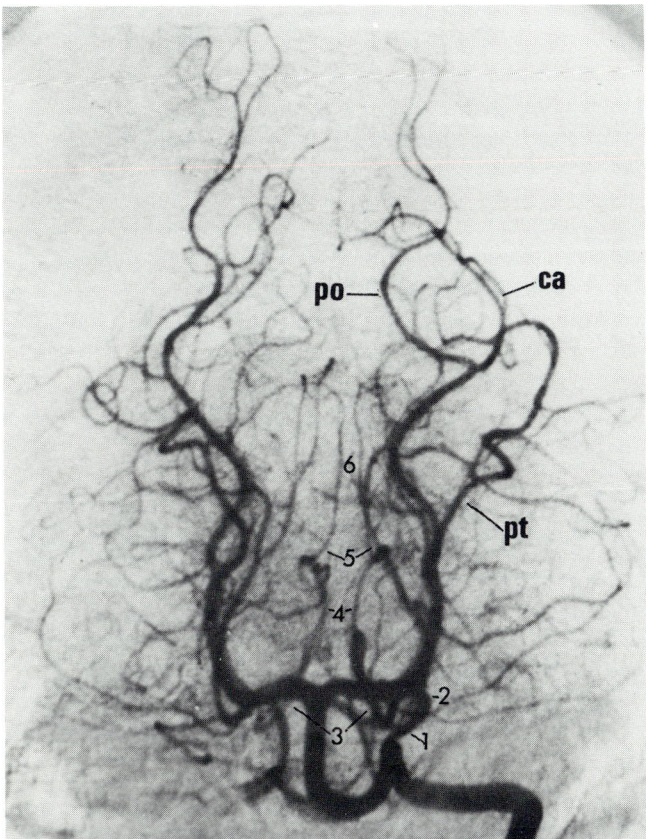

Fig. 4-8. Frontal projection. The anterior medullary segment (1), the lateral medullary segment (2), and the posterior medullary segments (3) of the left posterior inferior cerebellar artery are indicated. The posterior medullary and supratonsillar segments (4) show a medial convex curve due to the adjacent tonsils. The supratonsillar, retrotonsillar (5), and inferior vermian (6) segments approximate each other and lie in the midline.

The posterior temporal branch (pt) of the posterior cerebral artery extends laterally underneath the temporal lobe. The calcarine branch (ca) of the posterior cerebral artery supplies the calcarine cortex and is crossed by the parieto-occipital branch (po) which supplies the occipital lobe.

point.*[14] It is apparent that variations in the course of the PICA and its relationship to the fourth ventricle prevent any one measurement from being particularly useful. The position of Twining's point for the fourth ventricle and Sahlstedt's point for the aqueduct, however, are reliable and have stood the test of time.† Posterior fossa tumors usually displace both the fourth ventricle and aqueduct in similar directions. By constructing the fourth ventricle and aqueduct from Twining's and Sahlstedt's points (the average distance from the floor to the fastigium of the fourth ventricle we use is 12 ± 3 mm) and then relating the constructed fourth ventricle to the observed chorioidal point and the constructed aqueduct to the observed colliculo-central point obtained from the venous phase of the angiogram (see p. 82), valuable information about the displacement of these vessels can be obtained.

Twigs to the choroid plexus of the fourth ventricle can arise from the choroid arch. If these twigs are not recognized, a downward displacement of the fourth ventricle may be erroneously diagnosed. These vessels are best visualized by magnification and subtraction, but can also be recognized when

---

*Various measurements have been devised to evaluate the position of the choroidal point and vessels.

1. Huang and Wolf related the choroidal point to the anterior one-third point of a line connecting the anterior margin of the foramen magnum and the torcula.[14] In 50 presumably normal, adult angiograms, a vertical from the choroidal point to the line was on the average located from 1 mm anterior to 3 mm posterior to the anterior one-third point.

2. Megret constructed a line from the internal occipital protuberance to the end point of the basilar artery.[18] A perpendicular passing through the midpoint of this line was found to project over the choroidal twigs.

3. Wolf et al. related the cranial loop to Twining's line and found that a perpendicular from Twining's line passing through the cranial loop was situated between 53 and 59 percent of the length of Twining's line measured from the tuberculum sellae.[17]

4. Margolis and Newton utilized Twining's line and constructed a line from its midpoint to the posterior margin of the foramen magnum.[16] The apex of the choroid arch was situated within 7 mm in any direction of a point 2.5 cm below Twining's point along the constructed line in 60 normal angiograms magnified 2:1.

5. Peeters, in one study, found that the commencement of the choroid arch was always less than 1 cm posterior to Twining's point.[19] In another study, he found the choroid arch to be situated between 49 and 60 percent of the length of Twining's line measured from the tuberculum sellae.[20]

6. Belloni and DuBoulay described the blood supply to the choroid plexus as being derived from single or multiple choroidal arteries.[21] They defined the choroidal point as the point of origin of the largest choroidal artery from the PICA. The choroidal point was related to a line connecting the anterior margin of the foramen magnum and the internal occipital protuberance. In 77 percent of normal patients, a vertical from the choroidal point to the line was located between 33 and 43 percent of the length of the line.

†Sahlstedt stated that the junction of the first and middle thirds of a line joining the tip of the dorsum sellae through the lowest point of the aqueduct to the skull vault is situated immediately in front of the aqueduct.[22] Twining found that the midpoint of a line drawn between the tuberculum sellae and the internal occipital protuberance lay in the floor or just posterior to the floor of the fourth ventricle.[23]

pathologically enlarged.[18,24] In the semiaxial projection, the apex of the choroid arch averages a distance of 5 mm from the midline.[16]

The PICA continues backward over the superior pole of the tonsil and runs downward in the retrotonsillar fissure where it is known as the superior retrotonsillar segment. The artery then forms a loop convex inferiorly as it lies on the lower aspect of the inferior vermis, continuing around the copula pyramidus as the inferior vermian branch. The most anterior point of the curve of the pyramidal loop is called the copular point.* The loop may also be convex laterally on a frontal projection because the pyramid is wider and thicker than the other parts of the inferior vermis.[17] The terminal portion of the vermian branch curves around the tuber in the posterior cerebellar notch.[17] On each side, multiple inferior vermian branches are more frequent than a single branch.[27] Since the inferior vermis does not extend as far posteriorly as the cerebellar hemispheres, the vermian branches are projected parallel to, but at some distance from, the inner table of the skull on the lateral projection. The vermian branches may be up to 1 cm from the midline on a semiaxial projection.[16]

The tonsillohemispheric branch of PICA usually originates in the region of the cranial loop and runs inferiorly near the posterior margin of the tonsil (Figs. 4-4, 4-6, 4-13A). The vermian and tonsillohemispheric branches of PICA may be of varying size. Tonsillar branches extend anteriorly and hemispheric branches inferiorly and posteriorly from the tonsillohemispheric branch of PICA. The hemispheric branches run on the undersurface of the cerebellar hemisphere and, accordingly, project close to the occipital bone on the lateral projection.[17] The hemispheric branches anastomose with the hemispheric branches of the anterior inferior cerebellar artery and superior cerebellar artery.

Variations

Many of the variations of the vertebral artery are concerned with anomalous sites of origin. The most common variation is for the left vertebral artery to originate from the aorta between the left carotid and left subclavian arteries. This has been shown to occur in about 6 percent of cases.[28,29] The left vertebral artery has also been described as originating from the left common

*1. Leman and associates related the copular point to Twining's line and found that a perpendicular from Twining's line passing through the copular point was situated between 69 and 79 percent of the length of Twining's line measured from the tuberculum sellae.[25]

2. The measurement for the venous copular point as determined by Huang and co-workers can be used for the arterial copular point.[26] They related the copular point to the midpoint of a line joining the torcula and the anterior lip of the foramen magnum. They found that the copular point fell within a circle of 6 mm radius with its center 4 mm behind and below the midpoint.

3. Belloni and DuBoulay found that the copular point lay between 0 and 10 mm below a line drawn from the anterior lip of the foramen magnum to the internal occipital protuberance.[21]

carotid artery and also from the internal carotid artery.[30,31] This latter variation is called the pro-atlantal intersegmental artery when the communication is with the horizontal portion of the vertebral artery above the arch of C1.[30-33] If the communication with the vertebral artery is through a vessel which proceeds through the anterior condyloid foramen (hypoglossal canal) to the vertebral artery, bypassing the foramen magnum, the artery is called the primitive hypoglossal arteries, the proximal vertebral arteries are usually aplastic or hypoplastic.[30] Reported cases of origin of the vertebral artery from the external carotid artery in effect represent examples of the occipitovertebral anastomosis. The anastomosis is a normal communication between muscular branches of the vertebral artery and the occipital branch of the external carotid artery.[5,34]

The right vertebral artery has been described as originating from the right common carotid artery (associated with an anomalous origin of the right subclavian from the left side of the aortic arch). It can also originate from the left side of the aortic arch as the last branch.[30]

The left vertebral artery is larger than the right in 51 percent of cases (see Figs. 4-5, 4-8, 4-9), the right larger than the left in 41 percent (Figs. 4-17, 4-19), and the two vessels are of equal size in 8 percent (Fig. 4-2). Rarely, the vertebral artery may be absent on one side.[8]

Duplication of the vertebral artery has been reported.[3,8] This is most frequently seen involving the artery at the level of the atlantoaxial articulation, but it has also been seen involving the intracranial portion of the artery as well as the lower cervical portion (Figs 7-6B, 7-8).[8,35,36]

Non-union of the two vertebral arteries has been described.[37-39] In such cases, one vertebral artery terminates in PICA and the other in the basilar artery. A more frequent anomaly, however, is for the communication between the two vertebral arteries to be hypoplastic (Figs. 4-17, 4-19).

The PICAs are often asymmetrical in size and configuration (Figs. 4-4, 4-5, 4-16A, 4-18).[40,41] Variation of configuration is also frequent between the origin of PICA and the retrotonsillar segment. The positions of the copular point and the inferior vermian artery, however, are remarkably constant.

Either PICA may be entirely absent or hypoplastic, in which case the anterior inferior cerebellar artery (AICA) forms a large trunk, compensates for the absent or poorly developed artery, and supplies its territory. Under these circumstances, the usual loops of PICA may not be identifiable on a lateral film, and the appearances may simulate effacement of the loops by a vermian or hemispheric tumor (Figs. 4-9, 4-10). It is also possible to have a dominant PICA on one side and a dominant AICA on the other. Under these circumstances, the lateral film will show a combination of loops and smooth curves (Fig. 4-11). In one series, the PICA was absent on one or both sides in 24 percent of brains examined.[3]

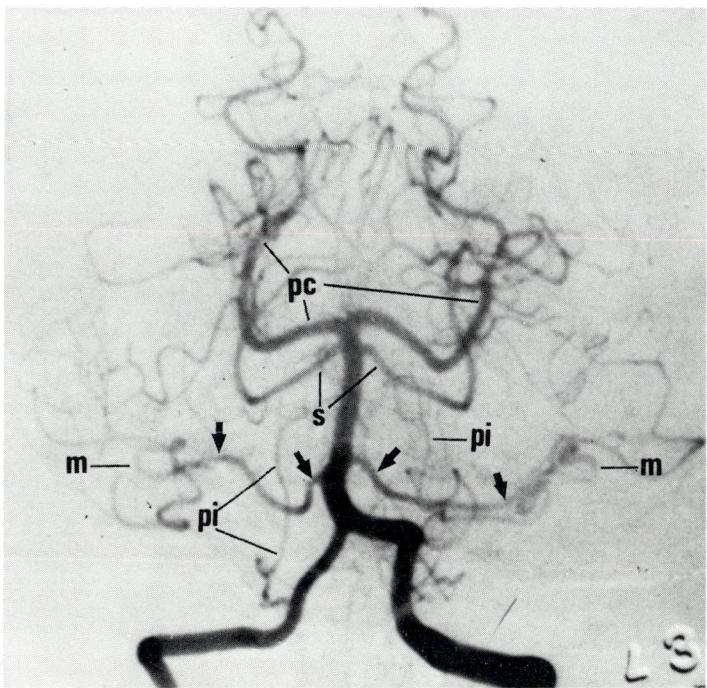

Fig. 4.9. Left vertebral angiogram, arterial phase, frontal projection: same case as Fig. 4-10. The left vertebral artery is larger than the right. The anterior inferior cerebellar arteries (arrows) are dominant and larger than the posterior inferior cerebellar arteries (pi). The anterior inferior cerebellar arteries can be identified both by their lateral course into the cerebellopontine angle cistern and by their characteristic loops (m). The superior cerebellar arteries (s) originate from the basilar artery immediately proximal to the posterior cerebral arteries (pc). The superior cerebellar arteries and the posterior cerebral arteries encircle the midbrain.

The caudal loop (lateral medullary segment) usually lies above the foramen magnum, but in 36 percent of normal cases, it may extend up to 20 mm below the foramen magnum (Fig. 4-12).[16] This appearance, therefore, should not be considered diagnostic of tonsillar herniation (see Chapter 8).

The relationship of PICA to the tonsil is subject to many variations.[15] While the artery often runs posteriorly above the tonsil as a supratonsillar segment, it may lie medial to the tonsil at a slightly lower level and is called a medial supratonsillar segment (Figs. 4-13A, B, 4-15, 4-18, 4-19). The artery, however, can also lie lateral to the tonsil as a lateral supratonsillar segment.[14] Under these circumstances, the artery on a semiaxial projection appears to be deviated laterally and to have a lateral convex curve instead of a

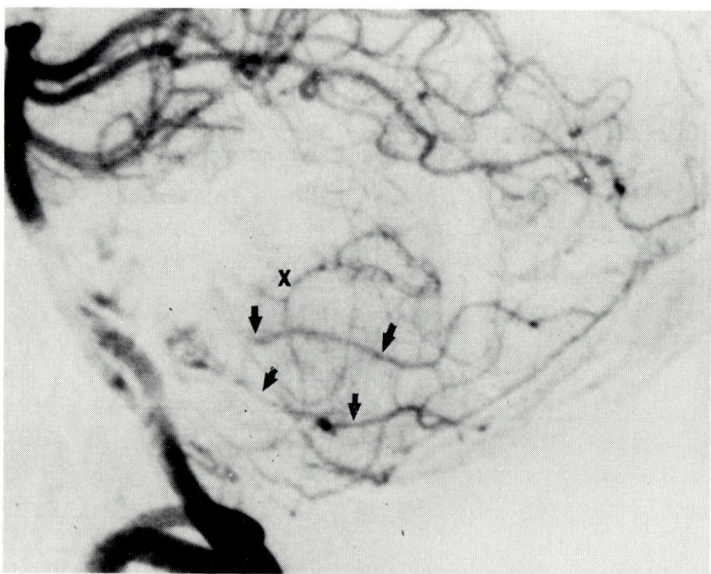

Fig. 4-10. Lateral projection. The anterior inferior cerebellar arteries (arrows) can be identified by their large undulant loops. The choroidal point (x) helps to identify the junction of the posterior medullary and supratonsillar segments of the posterior inferior cerebellar arteries.

medial convex curve (Figs. 4-14, 4-15). This appearance simulates fourth ventricular enlargement.[16] The artery can also lie adjacent to the inferior pole of the tonsil as a medial or lateral infratonsillar segment (Figs. 4-16A, B, 4-17, 4-20).

Instead of coursing posteriorly to the tonsil, the tonsillohemispheric branch may run inferiorly on the anterior aspect of the cerebellar tonsil.[14] This is a common variation (Figs. 4-7, 4-16A, 4-16B, 4-18, 4-19).

Other described variations of the PICA include:

  1. The PICA may supply only the tonsil and the inferior aspect of the cerebellar hemisphere. The vermian branches will then usually arise from the anterior inferior or the superior cerebellar vessels.[17]
  2. The PICA on one side may supply the opposite tonsil, the whole territory of the opposite PICA, or the opposite AICA (Fig. 4-21).[17]
  3. A small PICA on one side may frequently be associated with a large AICA on the same side and a large PICA on the opposite side.[42]

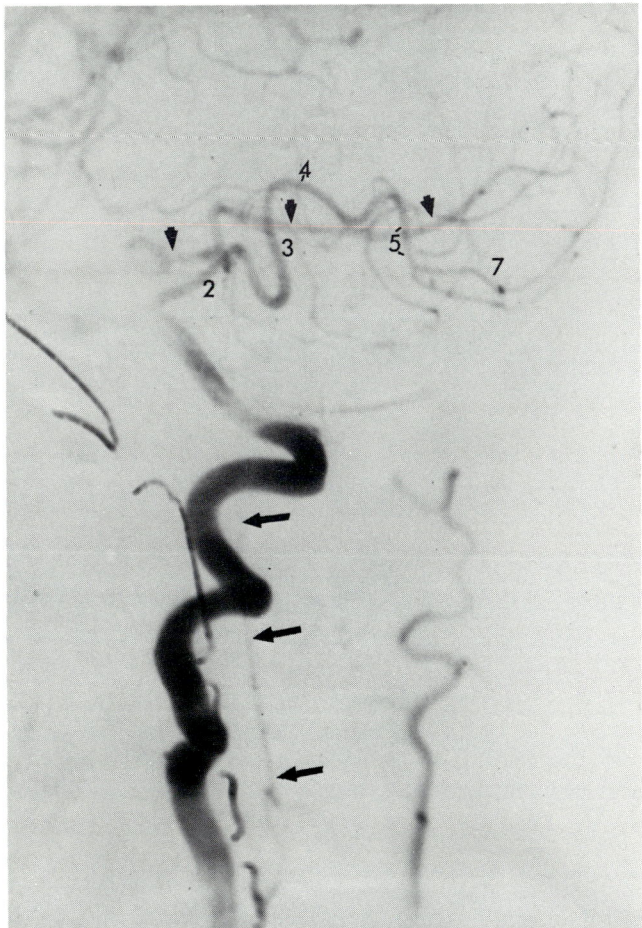

Fig. 4-11. Left vertebral angiogram, arterial phase, lateral projection. The typical loops of the posterior inferior cerebellar artery (2, 3, 4, 5, 7) are superimposed on the undulant curves of the anterior inferior cerebellar artery (short arrows). Note also the prominent anterior spinal artery (long arrows) on the anterior surface of the upper cervical cord. The large vessel posterior to the upper cervical spine is the ascending cervical branch of the thyrocervical trunk.

4. Both inferior vermian arteries may arise from PICA.
5. Occasionally the AICA and the superior cerebellar artery or the superior cerebellar artery alone can supply the whole cerebellar hemisphere.[27]

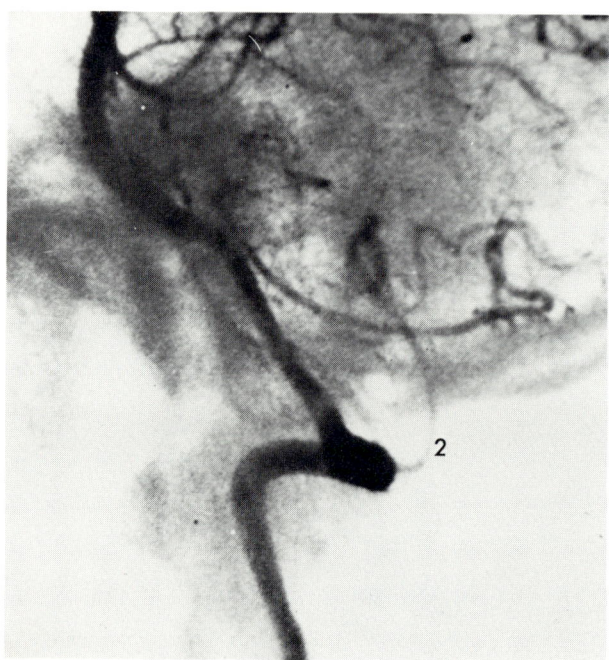

4-12. Left vertebral angiogram, arterial phase, lateral projection. The caudal loop (lateral medullary segment) (2) of the posterior inferior cerebellar artery extends inferiorly to the level of the arch of the atlas. This represents a normal variation.

BASILAR ARTERY

The basilar artery is formed by the union of the two vertebral arteries (see Fig. 4-2). It ascends in the pontine cistern along the anterior surface of the pons and terminates at the level of the dorsum sellae by bifurcating into the two posterior cerebral arteries. The artery becomes increasingly tortuous with age, in which case the apex of the artery may lie above and behind the dorsum sellae and thus indent the hypothalamus. In the semiaxial projection, the artery frequently makes a curve convex laterally. The convexity of the curve is usually contralateral to the dominant vertebral artery.[43, 44]

Branches

The branches of the basilar artery are the anterior inferior cerebellar artery, the pontine arteries, the labyrinthine artery (internal auditory artery), the superior cerebellar arteries, and the posterior cerebral arteries.[1]

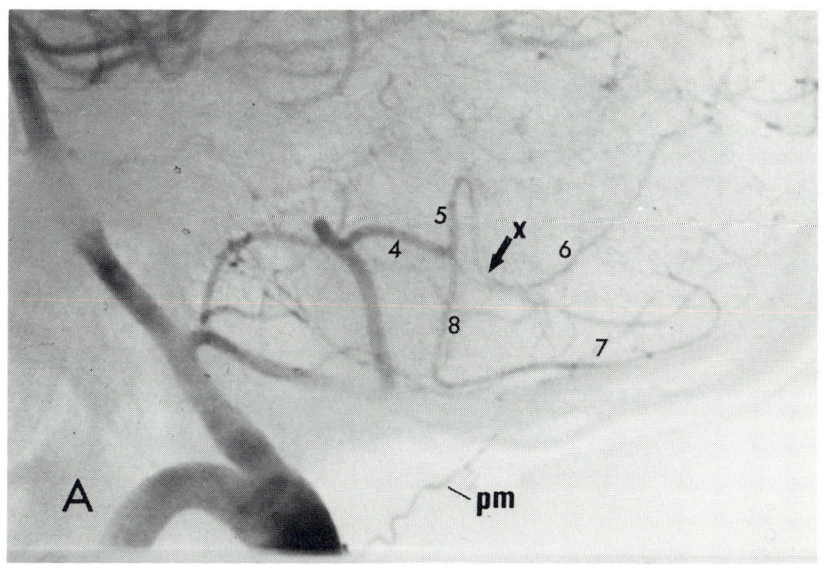

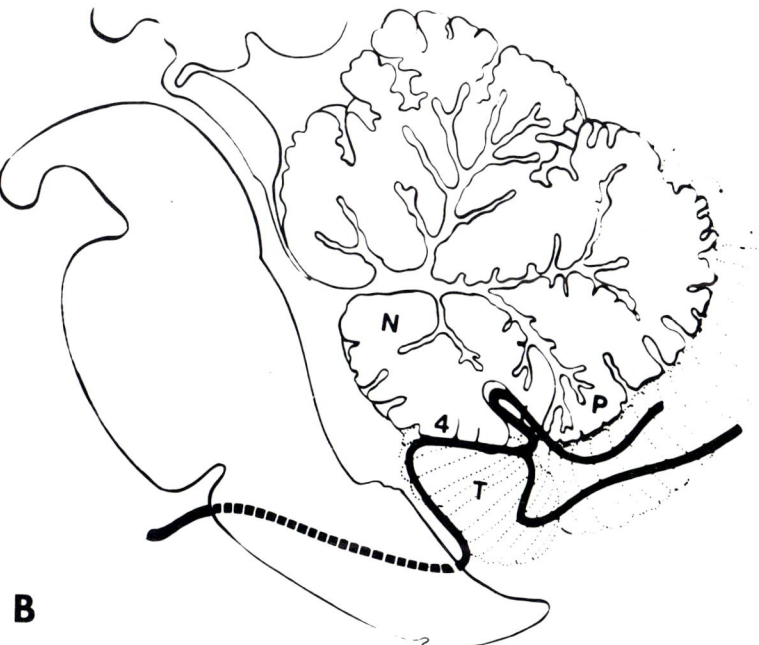

Fig. 4-13A,B. Left vertebral angiogram, arterial phase, lateral projection (4-13A) and line diagram (4-13B). The supratonsillar segment (4) lies slightly inferior to the upper pole. The remaining branches of the posterior inferior cerebellar artery (5, 6, 7, 8) are unremarkable. The copular point (x) is indicated. A posterior meningeal branch (pm) of the vertebral artery is seen originating from the third part of the vertebral artery on the angiogram. The nodulus (N), tonsil (T), and pyramis (P) are indicated on the diagram.

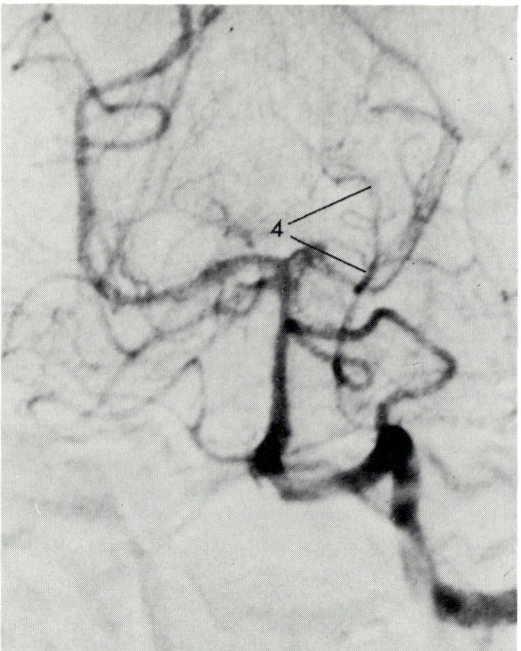

Fig. 4-14. Left vertebral angiogram, arterial phase, frontal projection. The supratonsillar segment (4) of the posterior inferior cerebellar artery lies lateral to the tonsil and, accordingly, has a lateral convex curve.

Anterior Inferior Cerebellar Artery

The anterior inferior cerebellar artery (AICA) usually originates from the middle or lower third of the basilar artery, extends laterally to cross the eighth nerve, and passes posteriorly around the pons to be distributed to the anterior aspect of the inferior surface of the cerebellum (Figs. 4-9, 4-22). In the majority of cases, the AICA originates as a single vessel from the basilar artery.[41] According to Atkinson, the AICA divides into medially and laterally directed branches, anastomosing with hemispheric branches of PICA and of the superior cerebellar artery.[45]

The course of AICA from the basilar artery to the region of the internal auditory meatus varies from straight to relatively tortuous.[41,46] The majority of cases exhibit an arterial loop in close relationship to the internal auditory canal (Figs. 4-9, 4-22). The loop was identified in 100 percent of a series of specimens and in 80 percent of a series of angiograms.[46,47] The arterial loop does not always involve the AICA. Mazzoni found the loop on the accessory

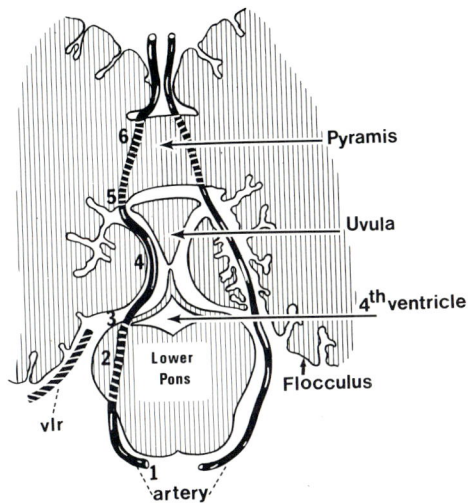

Fig. 4-15. Line diagram of a horizontal section through the pontomedullary junction. Note that the supratonsillar segment (4) of the posterior inferior cerebellar artery lies medial to the tonsil on the right side (reader's left) and lateral to the tonsil on the left side (reader's right). The anterior medullary (1), lateral medullary (2), posterior medullary (3), retrotonsillar (5), and inferior vermian (6) segments of the inferior vermian artery are demonstrated. The lateral medullary segment loops downward on the right side (reader's left) and is indicated by a dashed line; on the opposite side, it lies in the plane of the section. On the right side, the vein of the lateral recess (vlr) is seen between the flocculus and the posterolateral aspect of the medulla.

anterior inferior cerebellar artery (originating immediately distal to the AICA) in 17 percent of cases and on the posterior inferior cerebellar artery in 3 percent of cases.[47] Abrupt loops in the course of AICA are due in part to deviations around the seventh and eighth nerves. Different authors have studied the relationship of the AICA loop to the internal auditory canal and have found it to enter the canal in 40 percent of cases, to be at the orifice of the canal in 26 percent of cases, or to be unrelated to the canal in 34 percent of cases.[47,48]

Smaltino and associates, utilizing a different nomenclature, named the artery with a loop the cerebellolabyrinthine artery.[49] According to these authors, the cerebellolabyrinthine artery supplies the anterior surface of the cerebellum and the labyrinth. In 90 percent of cases, it is a branch of the anterior inferior cerebellar artery and, in 10 percent of cases, it is a branch of the basilar artery.

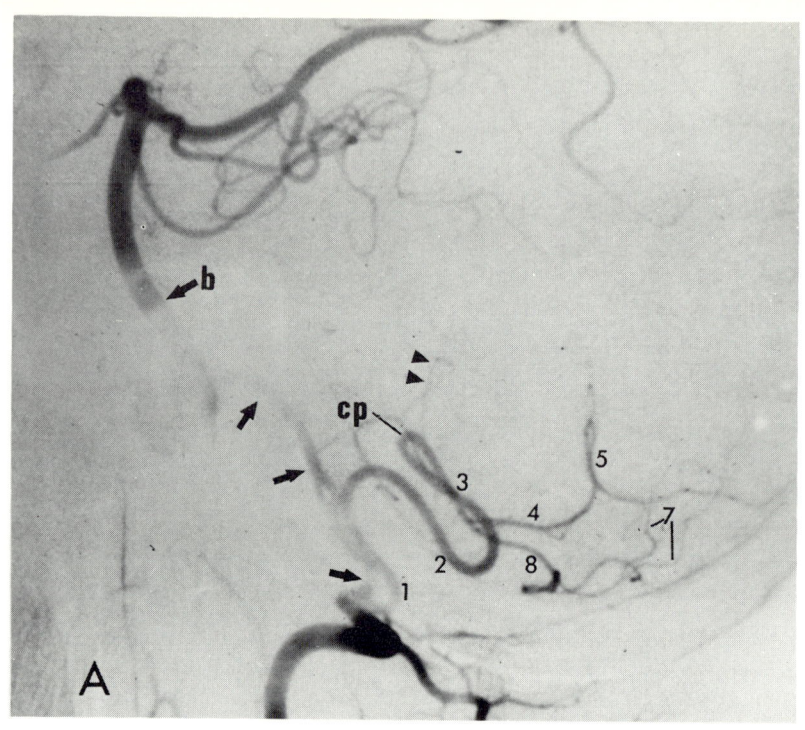
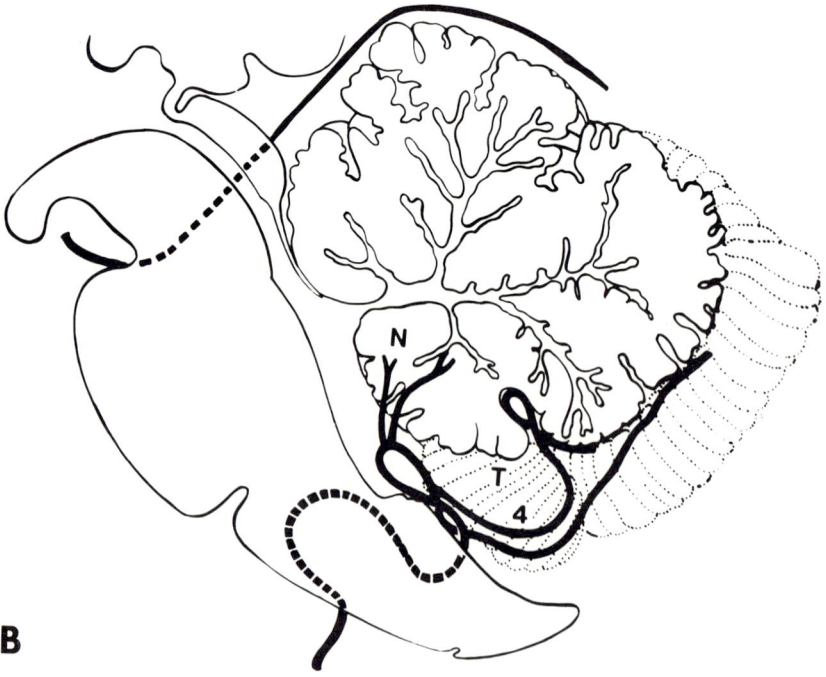

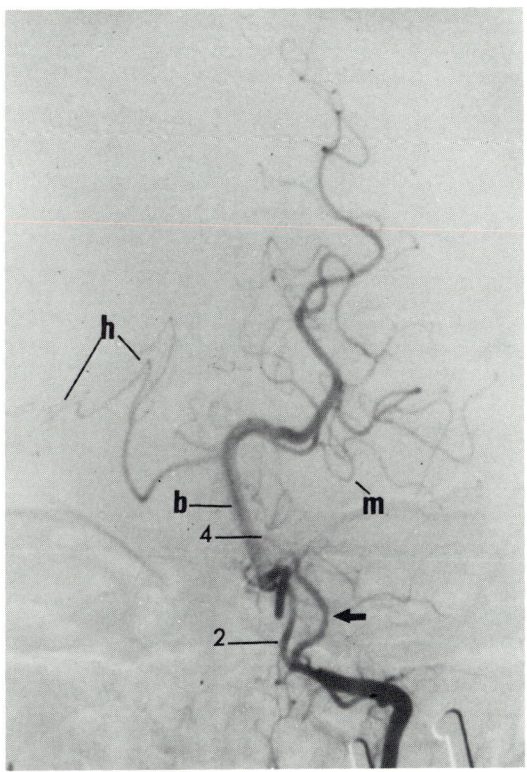

Fig. 4-17. Frontal projection. The hypoplastic left vertebral artery (arrow) is seen terminating in the normal-size basilar artery (b). The lateral medullary segment (2) of PICA is indicated. The infratonsillar segment (4) lies medial to the tonsil and can, accordingly, be called a medial infratonsillar segment. The marginal branch (m) of the superior cerebellar artery originates from the proximal part and the hemispheric branches (h) from the distal part of the ambient segment of the superior cerebellar artery.

Fig. 4-16A,B. Left vertebral angiogram, arterial phase, lateral projection (4-16A) and line diagram (4-16B): same case as Figs. 4-17 through 4-19. The fourth part of the vertebral artery (arrows) is hypoplastic but terminates in a normal-size basilar artery (b). The anterior medullary (1), lateral medullary (2), and posterior medullary (3) segments of the posterior inferior cerebellar artery are indicated. The tonsillar branch of PICA lies along the inferior surface of the tonsil and can, therefore, be considered as an infratonsillar segment (4). Small branches to the choroid plexus of the fourth ventricle (arrowheads) are seen arising from the choroidal point (cp). The tonsillohemispheric branch (8) of PICA originates from the infratonsillar segment. The retrotonsillar (5) and hemispheric branches (7) of PICA are indicated. The nodulus (N) and tonsil (T) are indicated on the diagram (Fig. 4-16B).

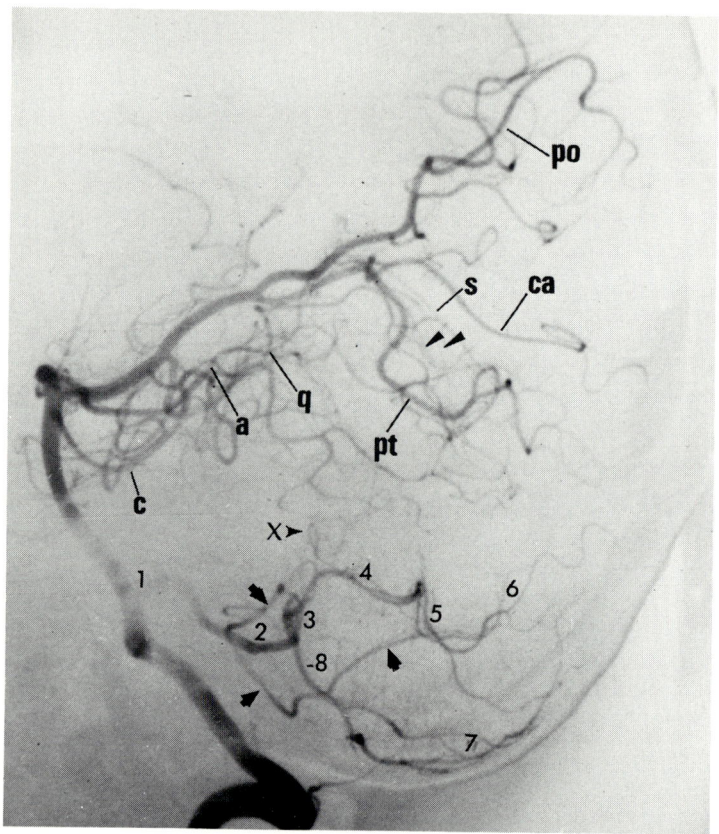

Fig. 4-18. Right vertebral angiogram, arterial phase, lateral projection. The anterior medullary (1), lateral medullary (2), and posterior medullary (3) segments of PICA are indicated. The tonsillohemispheric branch (8) originates from the posterior medullary segment and has hemispheric tributaries (7). A separate hemispheric branch (arrows) originates from the posterior medullary segment. Tiny vessels (X) originate from the choroidal point to supply the choroid plexus. The supratonsillar (4), retrotonsillar (5), and inferior vermian segments (6) of PICA are indicated. The supratonsillar segment (4) lies slightly below the apex of the tonsil. On the frontal view (4-19), it lies medial to the tonsil.

The crural segment (c) of the superior cerebellar artery has an inferior convex curve. The ambient (a) and quadrigeminal (q) segments are indicated. After curving over the top of the culmen, the superior vermian branch (s) descends along the declive. The parieto-occipital branch (po) projects as the highest, the calcarine branch (ca) the intermediate, and the posterior temporal branch (pt) the lowest of the posterior cerebral arterial branches. Note how the posterior temporal branch overlaps the hemispheric branches (arrowheads) of the superior cerebellar artery.

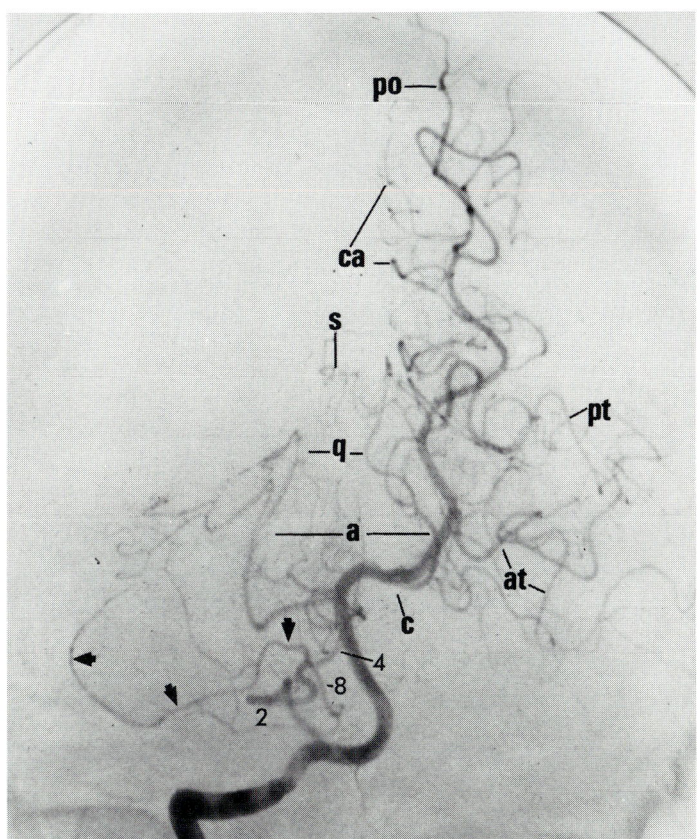

Fig. 4-19. Frontal projection. The right vertebral artery is the main supply to the basilar artery. The lateral medullary (2) and supratonsillar (4) segments of PICA are indicated. The tonsillohemispheric branch (8) originates from the posterior medullary segment together with a separate hemispheric branch (arrows) coursing laterally over the anterior (petrosal) surface of the cerebellar hemisphere. The crural segment (c) of the superior cerebellar artery has an inferior convex curve. The ambient segments (a) lie in the ambient cistern. The quadrigeminal segments (q) approximate each other behind the midbrain. The superior vermian segments (s) lie in the midline. The anterior temporal branch (at) and the posterior temporal branch (pt) of the posterior cerebral artery extend laterally. The calcarine branch (ca) extends medially and the parieto-occipital branch (po) posteriorly from a common origin, the internal occipital artery.

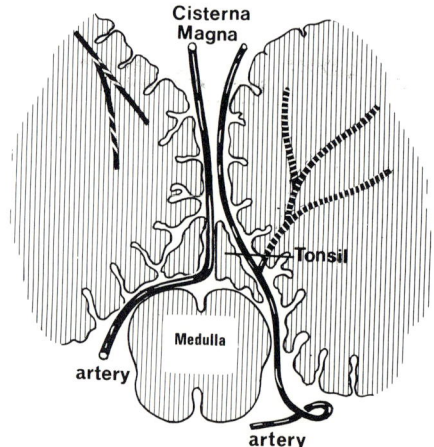

Fig. 4-20. Line diagram, horizontal section through the medulla. The posterior inferior cerebellar artery is seen coursing medial to the tonsil as a medial infratonsillar segment on the right side (reader's left) and as a lateral infratonsillar segment on the left side (reader's right).

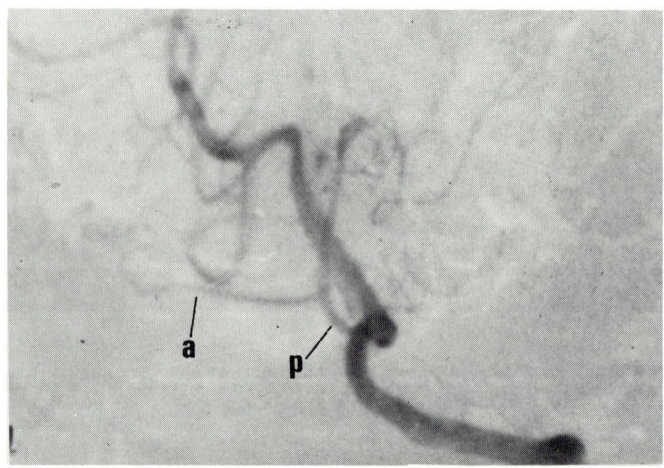

Fig. 4-21. Left vertebral angiogram, arterial phase, frontal projection. The right anterior inferior cerebellar artery (a) originates from the left posterior inferior cerebellar artery (p).

Normal Angiographic Anatomy of Posterior Fossa

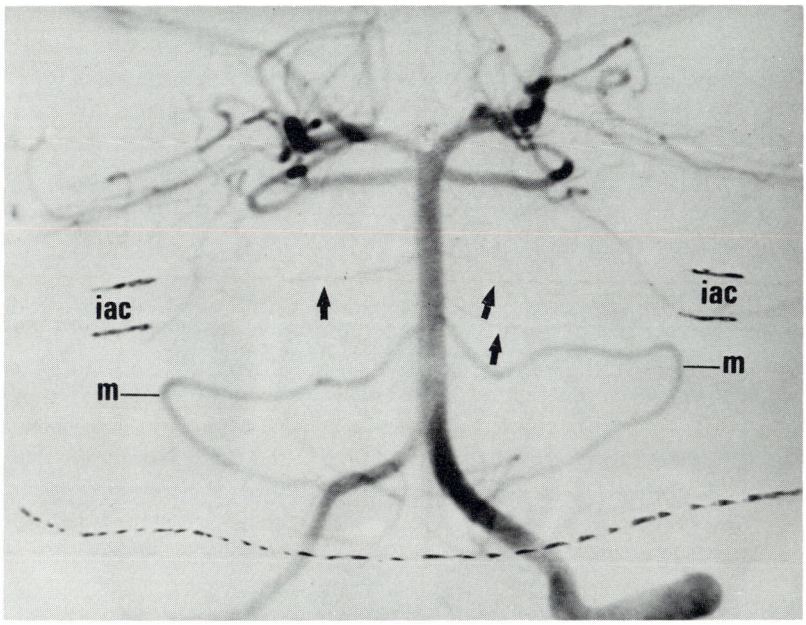

Fig. 4-22. Left vertebral angiogram, arterial phase, Caldwell projection. The anterior inferior cerebellar arteries extend laterally into the cerebellopontine angles and then exhibit characteristic loops (m), which in this case are seen to lie below the internal auditory canal (iac). Small, fine vessels are seen extending laterally (arrows) from the basilar artery and probably represent accessory anterior inferior cerebellar arteries rather than transverse pontine arteries.

Pontine Arteries

The pontine arteries are multiple and arise from the posterolateral surface (transverse pontine) and direct posterior surface (median pontine) aspects of the basilar artery.[3] The median pontine vessels lie on the ventral surface of the pons. Together with the pontine veins (see page 76), they outline the belly of the pons more accurately than the basilar artery that frequently swings laterally into the pontine cistern away from the surface of the pons. The transverse pontine vessels can usually be identified angiographically.[50] They are particularly well seen when pathologically enlarged (see Figs. 6-1, 6-5).

Labyrinthine Artery (Internal Auditory Artery)

The labyrinthine artery enters the internal auditory canal to supply the inner ear. Usually, this artery arises as a branch of the AICA, but, on occasion, it may arise directly from the basilar artery or from a branch of the

PICA.[3, 48, 51] According to Mazzoni, the internal auditory artery always arises from the arterial loop.[47] In 50 percent of cases, there are two or more internal auditory arteries.[47] Smaltino and co-workers found that the internal auditory artery originated from the cerebellolabyrinthine artery in 95 percent of cases, but in 5 percent of cases it originated from the basilar artery.[49] They identified the vessel angiographically in 73 percent of their angiograms.

Superior Cerebellar Arteries

The superior cerebellar arteries arise from the lateral aspects of the basilar artery immediately proximal to the basilar bifurcation near the upper border of the pons (Figs. 4-6 to 4-9, 4-18). Each superior cerebellar artery passes laterally, backward, and slightly downward over the upper surface of the pons, immediately below the oculomotor nerve. After winding around the cerebellar peduncle, the arteries reach the upper surface of the cerebellum where they supply the vermis and the upper surface of the cerebellar hemisphere.

Mani and associates[52] divided the superior cerebellar arteries into three main segments: interpeduncular-crural, ambient, and quadrigeminal. [These segments correspond to the prepontine, lateral pontine, and anterosuperior marginal segments as described by Huang et al. (Figs. 4-6, 4-7, 4-18, 4-19, 4-24).[53]] There are three major branches: marginal, hemispheric, and superior vermian (Figs. 4-17, 4-18, 4-23, 4-24).[52, 53]

MARGINAL ARTERY

The marginal artery originates from the ambient segment, courses forward, then posterolaterally.

HEMISPHERIC ARTERIES

The hemispheric arteries, usually two or three in number, originate from the ambient segment of the superior cerebellar artery and upon reaching the upper surface of the cerebellum fan out over the hemispheres.

SUPERIOR VERMIAN ARTERY

The superior vermian artery originates from the quadrigeminal segment of the superior cerebellar artery. Upon reaching the anterior aspect of the superior vermis, it runs upward and over the culminate lobe of the vermis (supraculminate segment).[53] Frequently, it anastomoses with the equivalent vessel on the opposite side. Terminally, it courses posteriorly over the vermis close to the midline. Two superior vermian branches may be present.

On the lateral projection of an angiogram, the interpeduncular-crural segment of the superior cerebellar artery often has a definite convex inferior

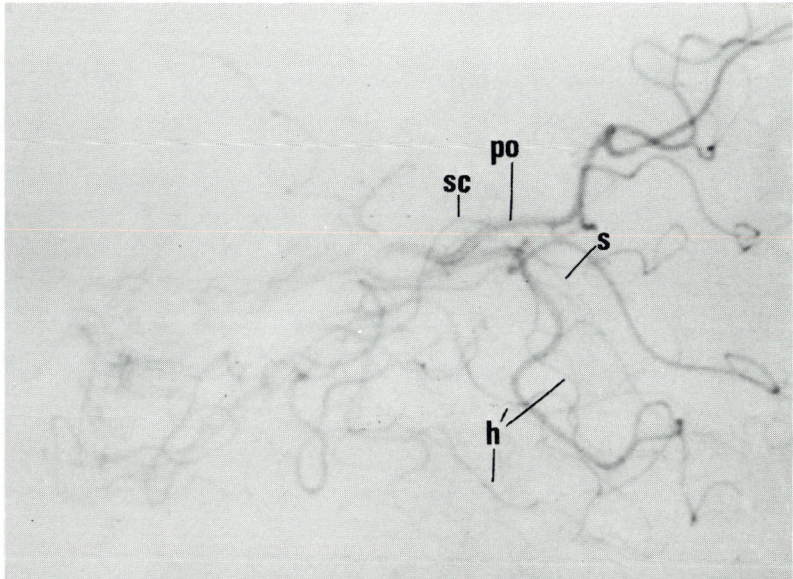

Fig. 4-23. Left vertebral angiogram, arterial phase, lateral projection (same patient as in 4-16A, one second later). The supraculminate segment (sc) of the superior cerebellar artery is seen as it courses over the culmen. This segment can project up to 9 mm above the occipital branch of the posterior cerebral artery (po). The superior cerebellar artery then descends over the declive as a superior vermian branch (s). The hemispheric branches (h) are parallel to the superior vermian branch and to each other.

curve (Figs. 4-6, 4-7, 4-18).[53] The hemispheric branches and the superior vermian branches have a stepladder-like arrangement, with the superior vermian branch forming the highest rung of the ladder (Fig. 4-23). The superior vermian branch (supraculminate segment) can project on a nonmagnified film up to 9 mm above the occipital branch of the posterior cerebral artery and still be within normal limits.[52] This anatomical arrangement is due to the configuration of the tentorium causing the occipital lobe to be inferolateral to the superior vermis.

In the semiaxial projection, the initial interpeduncular-crural segment lies inferior to the equivalent segment of the posterior cerebral artery, and the ambient segment of the superior cerebellar artery lies medial to the equivalent segment of the posterior cerebral artery (Figs. 4-9, 4-19). It appears as if the superior cerebellar artery crosses the posterior cerebral artery. The two superior vermian branches (one from each side) may, by anastomosing, complete a ring around the mesencephalon.

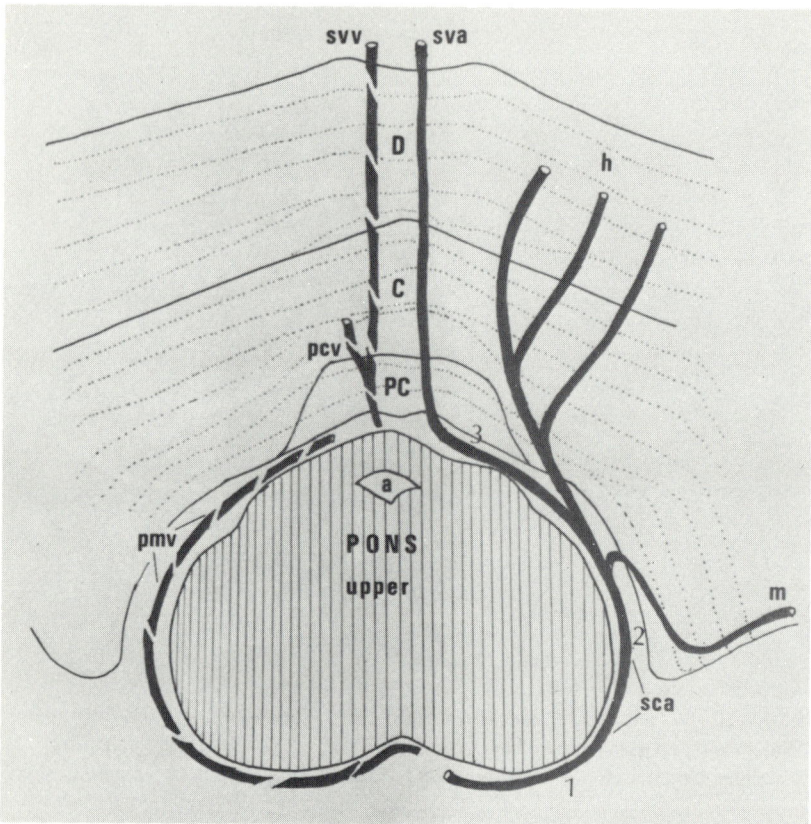

Fig. 4-24. Diagram of horizontal section through the upper pons. The crural (1), ambient (2), and quadrigeminal (3) segments of the superior cerebellar artery (sca) are seen as they encircle the upper pons. The terminal branches of the superior cerebellar artery consist of the marginal branch (m), hemispheric branches (h), and the superior vermian artery (sva). The superior vermian artery runs over the culmen (C) and the declive (D). On the reader's left the posterior mesencephalic vein (pmv) is indicated. The precentral cerebellar vein (pcv) is seen originating from a fissure in front of the precentral lobule (PC) of the cerebellum. The superior vermian vein (svv) is seen uniting with the precentral cerebellar vein. Often, however, the two veins empty separately into the great vein of Galen. The aqueduct is indicated (a).

Posterior Cerebral Arteries

The posterior cerebral arteries arise from the most rostral end of the basilar artery within the interpeduncular cistern (Figs. 4-7, 4-9). The posterior cerebral artery passes laterally around the cerebral peduncle in the ambient cistern to the posterolateral aspect of the midbrain. The initial segment of the posterior cerebral artery up to the site of the first branch (the posterior communicating artery) is called the interpeduncular or the P1 segment (by analogy with the A1 and M1 segments of the anterior and middle cerebral arteries respectively.)* As it encircles the midbrain, the posterior cerebral artery often makes a downward curve (convex inferiorly) (Fig. 4-7). The segment encircling the anterolateral aspect of the midbrain is called the crural segment. This segment leads to the ambient segment lying within the ambient cistern. The artery is contained within the tentorial incisura, and, as it extends dorsally, it becomes supratentorial to course under the inferior aspect of the temporal lobe. The two posterior cerebral arteries converge behind the brainstem as the quadrigeminal segments. The posterior cerebral artery terminates by supplying the medial aspect of the occipital lobe and the inferior surface of the temporal lobe.

The branches of the posterior cerebral artery are subdivided into cortical branches and penetrating branches.

CORTICAL BRANCHES

There are five main cortical branches: the anterior temporal, posterior temporal, parieto-occipital, and calcarine.[54] The posterior pericallosal artery is included as a cortical branch.

ANTERIOR TEMPORAL ARTERY

The anterior temporal artery (Figs. 4-19, 4-25) arises either as a single trunk or as multiple branches from the proximal ambient segment of the posterior cerebral artery.[54] The artery extends laterally and anteriorly beneath the hippocampal gyrus to supply the inferior aspect of the anterior portion of the temporal lobe. Here it can anastomose with the anterior temporal branches of the middle cerebral artery. In the lateral vertebral angiogram, the vessels are in the middle cranial fossa and are projected anterior to the basilar artery (Fig. 4-25).

POSTERIOR TEMPORAL ARTERY

The posterior temporal artery also arises from the ambient segment of the posterior cerebral artery and courses posteriorly and laterally along the hippocampal gyrus to supply the inferior aspect of the temporal and adjacent occipital lobe (Figs. 4-7, 4-8, 4-19).[54] The anterior and posterior

*The A1 segment of the anterior cerebral artery extends from its origin from the internal carotid to the origin of the first major branch, the anterior communicating artery. The M1 segment of the middle cerebral artery extends from its origin from the internal carotid artery to the first major cortical branch of the middle cerebral artery.

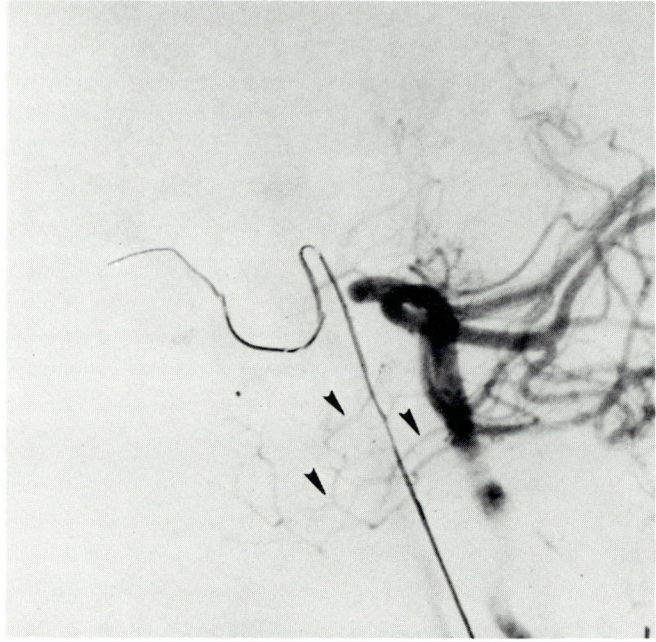

Fig. 4-25. Left vertebral angiogram, arterial phase, lateral projection. The anterior temporal branches (arrowheads) of the posterior cerebral artery lie anterior to the basilar artery.

temporal arteries can arise from a common trunk.[42] In the lateral vertebral angiogram, the posterior temporal artery courses posteriorly and inferiorly below the calcarine and parieto-occipital branches of the posterior cerebral artery (Figs. 4-7, 4-18). The vessels usually overlap the hemispheric branches of the superior cerebellar artery artery (Fig. 4-18).[28] In the semiaxial projection, the posterior temporal artery is the most lateral of the three posterior cortical branches (Figs. 4-8, 4-19).

PARIETO-OCCIPITAL AND CALCARINE ARTERIES

The parieto-occipital and calcarine arteries often originate from a common trunk, the internal occipital artery* (Figs. 4-7, 4-8, 4-18, 4-19).[28] The parieto-occipital artery, when it originates separately from the calcarine artery, arises from the posterior cerebral artery in either the ambient or quadrigeminal cistern. When it originates in common with the calcarine artery, it arises in the calcarine fissure on the medial surface of the occipital lobe.[54] The parieto-

---

*According to Taveras and Wood, the terminal division of the posterior cerebral artery are the posterior temporal artery and internal occipital artery.[28]

occipital artery courses over the cingulate gyrus and the medial portion of the parieto-occipital lobe. On the lateral angiogram, the parieto-occipital artery is the uppermost of the three posterior cortical branches (Figs. 4-7, 4-18). In the semiaxial projection, it is usually the most distally extending of the three branches (Figs. 4-8, 4-19).

The calcarine artery usually arises in the calcarine fissure and extends to the calcarine cortex. On the lateral angiogram, it lies between the posterior temporal and posterior occipital branches (Figs. 4-7, 4-18). On the semiaxial projection, while it originates lateral to the parieto-occipital artery, it crosses that artery to lie medial to the parieto-occipital branches (Figs. 4-8, 4-19).[54]

POSTERIOR PERICALLOSAL ARTERY

The posterior pericallosal artery originates either from the internal occipital branch of the posterior cerebral artery behind the midbrain, or directly from the posterior cerebral artery.[42, 55] It ascends behind and above the splenium of the corpus callosum (Fig. 4-26).[55] It forms a potential anastomotic ring with the pericallosal branch of the anterior cerebral artery.[28]

PENETRATING BRANCHES

The penetrating branches of the posterior cerebral artery can be divided into thalamoperforating arteries, quadrigeminal and geniculate body arteries, and posterior choroidal arteries. The branches supply the basal ganglia, thalami, choroid plexus, pineal area, and tectum.

ANTERIOR AND POSTERIOR THALAMOPERFORATING ARTERIES

Westberg describes an anterior thalamoperforating artery originating from the posterior communicating artery,* and posterior thalamoperforating arteries originating from the apex of the basilar artery and the P1 segment of the posterior cerebral artery.[56] The arteries extend obliquely upward and backward, lateral to the third ventricle, into the hypothalamus (Figs. 4-26, 4-27).[57]

QUADRIGEMINAL AND GENICULATE BODY ARTERIES

The quadrigeminal artery arises from the crural segment of the posterior cerebral artery, runs parallel to the medial posterior choroidal artery, and terminates by supplying the colliculi. The geniculate body arteries originate from the ambient segment of the posterior cerebral artery and supply the posterior half of the thalamus.[42] Since both the quadrigeminal and geniculate

---

*The posterior communicating artery forms a communication between the posterior cerebral artery and the internal carotid artery.

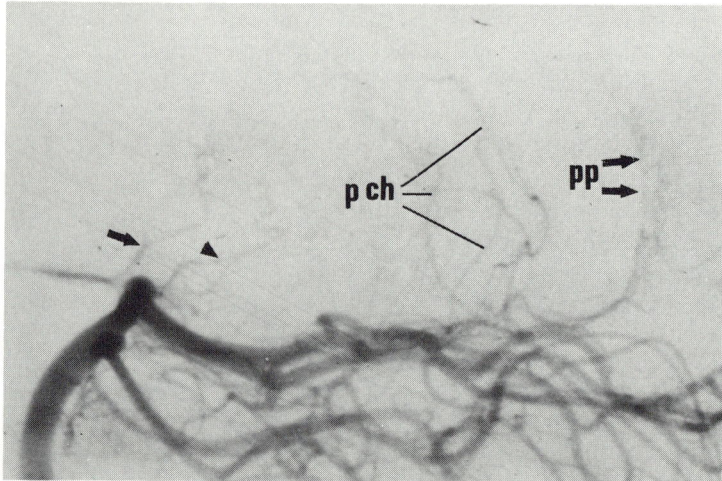

Fig. 4-26. Left vertebral angiogram, arterial phase, lateral projection. The posterior pericallosal artery (pp) originates from the posterior cerebral artery behind the midbrain. The artery extends superiorly behind and then above the splenium of the corpus callosum. Anteriorly, the anterior thalamoperforating artery (arrow) originates from the posterior communicating artery, and the posterior thalamoperforating artery (arrowhead) from the apex of the basilar and proximal posterior cerebral arteries. The posterior choroidal arteries (pch) are seen between the posterior pericallosal and thalamoperforating arteries.

arteries closely parallel the posterior choroidal arteries, their angiographic identification is very difficult.

POSTERIOR CHOROIDAL ARTERIES

The posterior choroidal arteries (Fig. 4-26) are divided into medial and lateral branches. The medial branch originates from the interpeduncular-crural segments of the posterior cerebral artery and then curves around the midbrain with the posterior cerebral artery to ascend to the pineal region and then ends in the tela choroidea of the roof of the third ventricle. On a lateral angiogram, it often adopts a figure "3" configuration with double anterior concave curves (Fig. 4-27). In the region of the pineal gland, the artery may run lateral to or posterior to the gland before extending anteriorly in the tela choroidea of the roof of the third ventricle.[58,59] The lateral posterior choroidal arteries, which are usually multiple, originate from either the interpeduncular-crural or ambient segments of the posterior cerebral artery lateral to the midbrain and then ascend to enter the choroidal fissure where they terminate in supplying the choroid plexus of the temporal horn and trigone with branches to the tela choroidea (Fig. 4-28). On a lateral angiogram, the curve of the lateral posterior

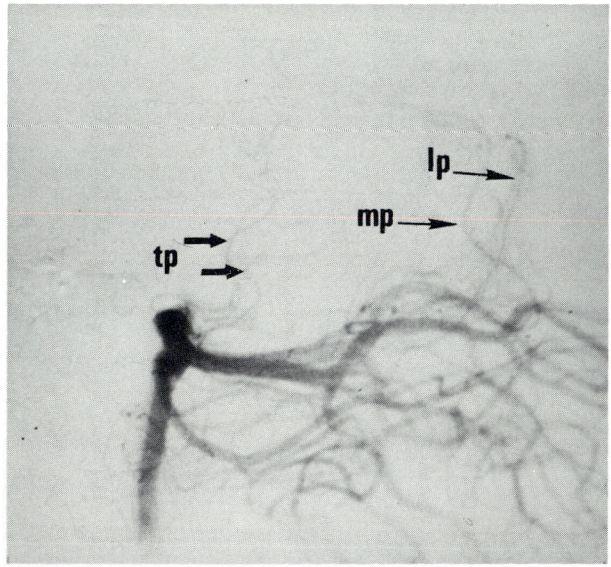

Fig. 4-27. Left vertebral angiogram, arterial phase, lateral projection. The medial posterior choroidal artery (mp) has the configuration of a "3" which distinguishes it from the lateral posterior choroidal artery (lp). The thalamoperforating arteries (tp) anteriorly have a typical sinuous configuration.

choroidal artery lies posterior to that of the medial posterior choroidal artery and, accordingly, has a wider, more even sweep around the pulvinar of the thalamus (Fig. 4-27).[59] According to Löfgren, the lateral posterior choroidal artery lies between 29 and 46 mm posterior to the apex of the basilar artery at approximately the level of the trigone, as measured on films utilizing a focus-film distance of 75 cm.[58]

Variations

Variations of the basilar artery are rare. Areas of duplication can occur involving part of or the whole length of the artery.[36, 38, 60]

The anterior inferior cerebellar arteries can vary considerably in size and, therefore, in importance of vascular supply. Frequently, there is also a difference between the two sides. Variations in size are frequently in inverse proportion to the size of the posterior inferior cerebellar artery.[41, 45] Accessory anterior inferior cerebellar arteries originating from the basilar artery may also occur.[45]

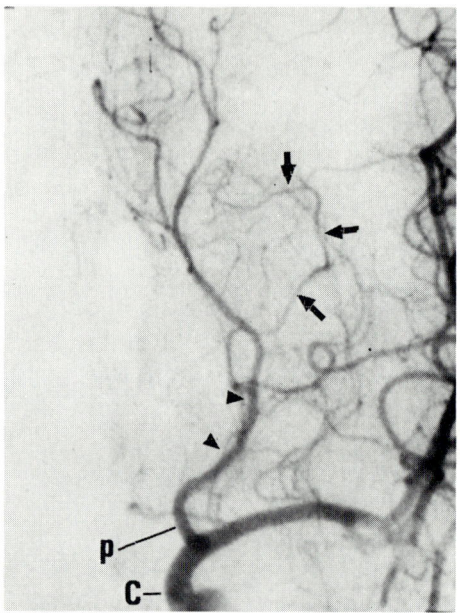

Fig. 4-28. Left carotid angiogram, arterial phase, frontal projection. The left posterior cerebral artery (arrowheads) originates from the internal carotid artery (C) through a large posterior communicating artery (p). The lateral posterior choroidal artery (arrows) is seen originating from the ambient segment of the posterior cerebral artery. It has a typical convex lateral curve as it sweeps around behind the pulvinar of the thalamus to supply the choroid plexus in the lateral ventricles.

The anterior inferior cerebellar artery can supply the choroid plexus of the lateral recess of the fourth ventricle.[42] Not infrequently, the internal auditory artery will originate from the accessory anterior inferior cerebellar artery.[47]

The superior cerebellar artery may be double for all or part of its course. This was observed in 31 percent of a series 150 brains[3] and in 28 percent of a series of 100 angiograms.[52] Bilateral duplication of the superior cerebellar artery was seen in 8 percent of the 100 angiograms.

In 30 percent of brains, the posterior cerebral artery originating from the internal carotid artery by a large posterior communicating artery remains as a major cortical branch on one or both sides (see Fig. 4-28).[61, 62] In these cases, the P1 segment of the posterior cerebral artery is reduced in caliber or absent.

Congenital anastomoses between the carotid and basilar arteries may occur. These include the persistent trigeminal artery, the otic artery, and the hypoglossal artery.[30] When these anastomoses persist, the vertebral arteries are usually hypoplastic or absent.

MENINGEAL ARTERIES

The posterior fossa is completely lined by dura except for the foramen magnum inferiorly and the tentorial incisura superiorly. The meningeal arteries can be divided into inferior, anterosuperior, and lateral groups.

INFERIOR GROUP

The meningeal branches of the vertebral artery supply the dura over the convexity of the inferior cerebellar hemisphere and the dura surrounding the foramen magnum. There are two major divisions arising from the extracranial vertebral artery—a posterior and an anterior branch.[63]

POSTERIOR BRANCH

The posterior branch originates from the vertebral artery above the arch of the atlas and enters the skull via the lateral portion of the foramen magnum. The branch ramifies between the bone and dura mater and supplies the falx cerebelli (Figs. 4-13A, 5-18, 5-19, 8-16, 8-18).[63, 64] It has a tortuous extracranial, but a straight intracranial course where it is seen approximately in the midline in the semiaxial projection. On the lateral projection, it lies a few millimeters from the bony attachment of the falx to the occipital bone. Not infrequently, the artery extends beyond the tentorium into the falx cerebri. In normal angiograms, the posterior branch can be seen arising from the vertebral arteries in 30 to 40 percent of cases.[63, 65] It may arise from the external occipital artery or the ascending pharyngeal artery.[64, 66, 67]

ANTERIOR BRANCH

The anterior meningeal branch of the vertebral artery originates from the vertebral artery immediately below its first bend at the level of the axis (Figs. 4-3, 5-2A, B, 5-4). After entering the spinal canal, it courses upward, lies anterior and close to the midline, and supplies the dura at the foramen magnum.[68] On angiograms, the artery can be identified in 40 to 50 percent of normal angiograms.[63, 68] It always projects anterior to the anterior spinal artery in a lateral projection.[68]

ANTEROSUPERIOR GROUP

The meningeal branches to the dura over the clivus and the tentorium originate from the meningohypophyseal trunk which is a branch of the cavernous carotid artery. Detailed anatomical studies have been presented by Schnürer and Stattin, McConnell, and Parkinson.[69-71] There are three subdivisions: a tentorial artery, a dorsal meningeal (dorsal clival) artery, and an inferior hypophyseal artery. Branches of the meningohypophyseal trunk make direct arterial anastomoses with the middle meningeal and the accessory meningeal arteries, and, often, the main blood supply to the tentorium and petrous dura is derived from these branches.[72]

TENTORIAL ARTERY

The tentorial artery runs about 5 mm from the free margin of the tentorium and then extends for a short distance up the falx cerebri.

DORSAL MENINGEAL ARTERY

The dorsal meningeal artery (see Fig. 5-6A) leaves the meningohypophyseal trunk in a posteroinferomedial direction to supply the dura over the clivus.[64] It anastomoses with the contralateral artery and with the meningeal branch of the vertebral artery.

INFERIOR HYPOPHYSEAL ARTERY

The inferior hypophyseal artery supplies the posterior lobe of the pituitary gland.

LATERAL GROUP

Meningeal supply to the dura over the cerebellar convexity is derived from a number of sources. The following branches all can provide blood supply to this area.[1, 64]

MENINGEAL BRANCH OF EXTERNAL OCCIPITAL ARTERY*

The meningeal branch of the occipital artery ascends with the internal jugular vein to enter the skull through the jugular foramen and condyloid canal and through an emissary foramen behind the mastoid process.[1] The branch supplies the dura mater over the lateral surface of the cerebellum (see Fig. 8-24A).

POSTERIOR BRANCH OF MIDDLE MENINGEAL ARTERY*

The posterior branch of the middle meningeal artery supplies the parietooccipital dura, but can also supply the dura over the lateral surface of the cerebellum (see Fig. 8-24A). It can also supply the dura adjacent to the trigeminal ganglia.[1]

RECURRENT BRANCHES OF MIDDLE MENINGEAL ARTERY*

These branches are derived from the middle meningeal artery and supply the dura over the posteriorsuperior surface of the temporal bone.

MENINGEAL BRANCHES OF ASCENDING PHARYNGEAL ARTERY*

The meningeal branches of the ascending pharyngeal artery enter the cranium through either the jugular foramen, the foramen lacerum, or, on occasions, through the hypoglossal canal.[1] These vessels supply the meninges lining the posterior surface of the petrous bone and the cerebellopontine angle.[64]†

The lateral group of meningeal arteries is also difficult to see if not pathologically enlarged (see Fig. 5-5A).

CERVICOVERTEBRAL VEINS

The cervicovertebral venous system is divided into five sets of veins which, separately or together, aid in the venous drainage from the posterior fossa.

JUGULAR VEIN

The jugular vein constitutes the main drainage system from the cranium. It forms a continuation of the sigmoid sinus which leaves the skull through the jugular foramen as a slight venous dilatation called the jugular sinus. At the point of junction of the jugular sinus and jugular vein is the inferior petrosal sinus which drains the blood from the cavernous sinus (Fig. 4-29).

VERTEBRAL VEIN

The vertebral vein is formed in the supoccipital triangle at the back of the neck by tributaries from the suboccipital venous plexuses and by small muscular veins. The vertebral vein enters the foramen in the transverse process of the atlas and then descends as a venous plexus surrounding the vertebral artery.[1] The plexus ends as a single trunk emerging from the foramen transversarium of either the fifth or sixth cervical vertebra to empty into the brachiocephalic vein near its origin. The vertebral vein communicates with the sigmoid and inferior petrosal sinuses through the suboccipital plexus.[73]

*The external occipital, middle meningeal, and ascending pharyngeal arteries are branches of the external carotid artery.
†"The tympanum is partially supplied by the tympanic branch of the ascending pharyngeal artery."[1]

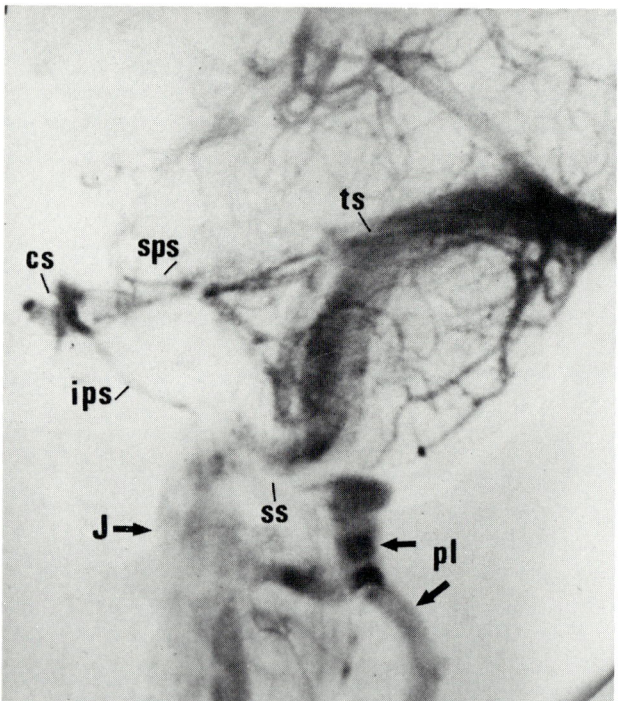

Fig. 4-29. Left vertebral angiogram, venous phase, lateral projection. The internal jugular vein (J) constitutes the main venous pathway from the brain. The inferior petrosal sinus (ips) communicates between the cavernous sinus (cs) and the jugular vein. The superior petrosal sinus (sps) lies along the tentorial attachment to the petrous bone anterolaterally and drains blood back to the transverse sinus (ts) which communicates with the jugular vein via the sigmoid sinus (ss). A large occipital vein (p1) is seen communicating freely with the jugular vein and sigmoid sinus.

SUBOCCIPITAL VENOUS PLEXUS

A rich venous plexus is present in the suboccipital area freely communicating superiorly with the basal venous sinuses through the anterior condylar vein and inferiorly with the vertebral vein. On angiography, a plexus of veins can often be seen in the suboccipital triangle, contributing to a rich anastomosis between the many veins in this area. According to Backmund and associates, these veins, which can be visualized in 64 percent of normal carotid angiograms, represent a usual and frequent drainage pathway for the cerebral circulation (Fig. 4-29).[74]

CERVICAL EPIDURAL VENOUS SYSTEM

The cervical epidural venous system lines the inner surface of the spinal canal. The system communicates superiorly with the suboccipital plexus and the basal venous sinuses. Inferiorly, there is a communication with the thoracic epidural veins. Dilenge and Perey consider that the main drainage channel for blood from the cranium is the epidural venous system in the erect position and the jugular veins in the supine position.[75]

Théron and Djindjian have successfully demonstrated the vertebral and epidural veins by catheterization of both the anterior condyloid and vertebral veins.[73] Their approach consisted of the retrograde catheterization of the femoral vein using the Seldinger method.

SPINAL CORD VEINS

Spinal veins lying on the anterior and posterior aspects of the spinal cord were frequently identified by Gabrielsen and co-workers.[11] They claimed that the anterior border of the upper cervical cord could usually be better localized during the arterial rather than venous phase, whereas the reverse was true for the posterior border. The anterior spinal vein communicates with the ponto-mesencephalic vein (see p. 76).

POSTERIOR FOSSA VEINS

According to Huang and Wolf, the veins of the posterior fossa may be divided into anterior (petrosal), superior (Galenic), and posterior (tentorial) groups.[76]

Anterior (Petrosal) Group[77]

The anterior group drains the anterior part of the brainstem and the cerebellum and empties, ultimately, into the superior and inferior petrosal sinuses. The main route for drainage is the petrosal vein which lies in the cerebellopontine angle. The following veins generally drain into the petrosal vein: ponto-mesencephalic vein, brachial veins, superior and inferior hemispheric veins, cerebellomedullary vein, and vein of the lateral recess of the fourth ventricle.

Ponto-mesencephalic Vein

The ponto-mesencephalic vein outlines the floor of the hypothalamus, the anterior border of the mesencephalon, and the anterior margin of the pons (Figs. 4-30, 4-31).[77,78] In effect, therefore, it outlines the interpeduncular and pontine cisterns. It can be divided into mesencephalic and pontine segments. The pathway of drainage is inferolaterally to the petrosal vein, although alternative pathways through the basal vein of Rosenthal or the posterior mesencephalic vein to the great vein of Galen are possible (see variations). A transverse pontine vein communicates between the ponto-mesencephalic vein and the petrosal vein. Since the pontine segment of the ponto-mesencephalic vein lies in the midline on the anterior margin of the pons, it delineates the pons more accurately than the basilar artery which frequently does not follow the anterior margin of the pons.

Brachial Veins

The brachial veins lie on the brachium pontis. They drain anterolaterally to join the petrosal vein. Often, they form communications through the lateral anastomotic mesencephalic vein with the posterior mesencephalic vein which drains posteriorly, superiorly, and medially to the great vein of Galen (Figs. 4-30, 4-31, 4-32).[77]

Superior and Inferior Hemispheric Veins

The superior and inferior hemispheric veins drain the superior and inferior surfaces of the cerebellar hemisphere. Typically, the superior hemispheric veins course anteriorly and inferiorly around the cerebellar hemispheres before draining into the petrosal vein and, therefore, have arcuate convex lateral configurations on a semiaxial projection. While the inferior hemispheric veins most often drain forward into the petrosal sinuses, they may drain backward into the posterior (tentorial) group of veins (Figs. 4-30, 4-31, 4-32, 4-34).[77]

Vein of Lateral Recess of Fourth Ventricle

The vein originates close to the lateral recess of the fourth ventricle in the posterolateral fissure which is bordered by the brachium pontis, inferomedial aspect of the cerebellum, and upper medulla. The vein extends inferolaterally to unite with the petrosal vein (Figs. 4-33, 4-34, 4-35).[79,80]

Normal Angiographic Anatomy of Posterior Fossa

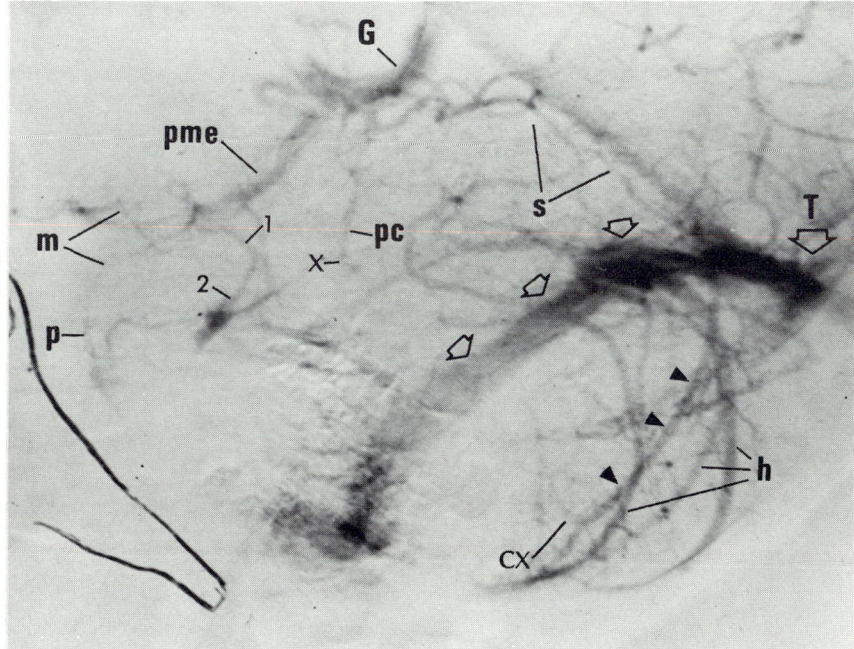

Fig. 4-30. Left vertebral angiogram, venous phase, lateral projection. The ponto-mesencephalic vein can be divided into mesencephalic (m) and pontine (p) segments that outline the anterior margin of the pons and the interpeduncular cistern. The posterior mesencephalic vein (pme) surrounds the midbrain and drains blood posteriorly to the great vein of Galen (G). A communication is present between the posterior mesencephalic vein and the petrosal vein through a brachial vein (2) and a lateral anastomotic vein (1). The precentral vein (pc) in the precentral fissure has a typical convex knee (X) at the colliculo-central point. A superior vermian vein (s) is seen outlining the declive. Hemispheric veins (h) can be recognized by their curvilinear configurations and their typical termination in the transverse sinus (unlabeled open arrows). The inferior vermian vein (arrowheads) terminates posteriorly in the region of the torcula (T). Inferiorly, it has a typical convex curve making the copula pyramidal point (CX).

Cerebellomedullary vein

The cerebellomedullary vein runs superiorly on the lateral border of the medulla to end in the petrosal vein.[77]

Petrosal Vein

The petrosal vein lies within the cerebellopontine angle and drains into the superior petrosal sinus (Figs. 4-32, 4-34, 4-35, 4-38). Characteristically, in the

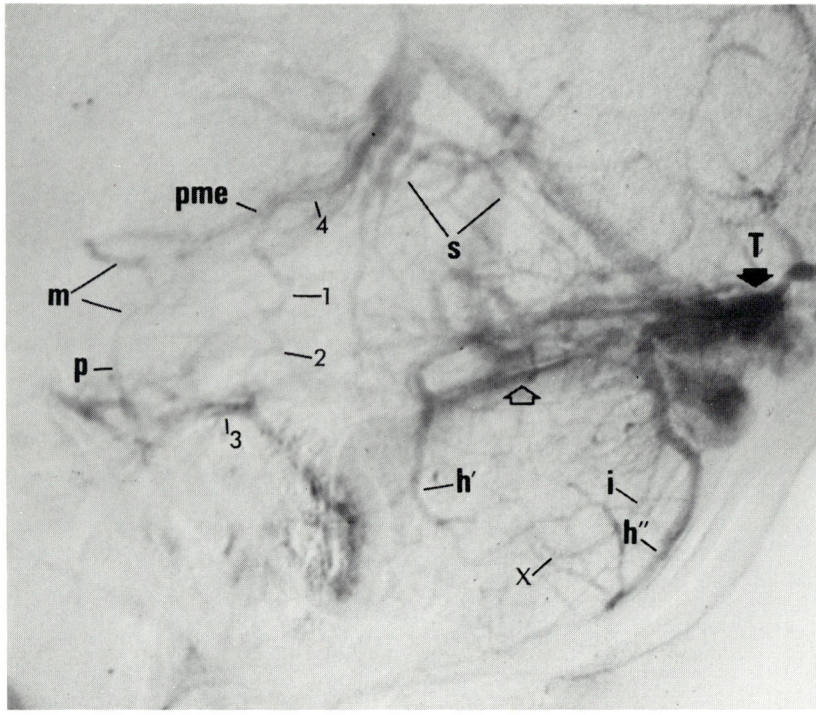

Fig. 4-31. Left vertebral angiogram, venous phase, lateral projection. The mesencephalic (m) and pontine (p) segments of the ponto-mesencephalic vein are seen anteriorly. Through the brachial vein (2) and the lateral anastomotic vein (1), the left posterior mesendephalic vein (4) communicates with the petrosal vein (3). The right posterior mesencephalic vein (pme) extends farther anteriorly than the left and communicates with the mesencephalic portion of the ponto-mesencephalic vein. A well-defined supraculminate segment (s) of the superior vermian vein can be identified. An inferior hemispheric vein (h') terminates in the transverse sinus (open arrow). A second inferior hemispheric vein (h") atypically terminates in the torcula (T). A small inferior vermian vein (i) can be recognized by the typical inferior convex curve marking the copula pyramidal point (x).

semiaxial projection, the vein can be recognized by its typical course extending inferolaterally at about 45° to unite with the superior petrosal sinus immediately above the internal auditory meatus.[81, 82] Opacification of the petrosal vein in the normal case depends largely on whether the posterior inferior cerebellar artery is opacified.[81, 82] Accordingly, in posterior fossa angiography, it is always advisable to inject the vertebral artery on the side of a suspected lesion. If, during angiography, adequate reflux down the opposite vertebral artery is obtained, both petrosal veins will be opacified.

Normal Angiographic Anatomy of Posterior Fossa

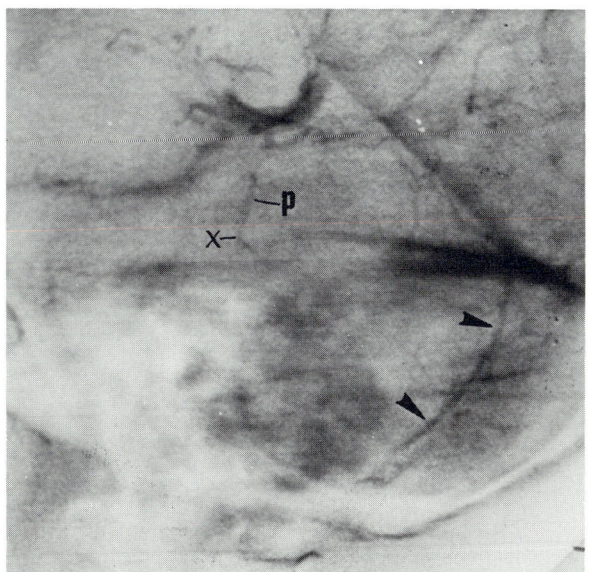

Fig. 4-32. Frontal projection. The right posterior mesencephalic vein (pme) makes a characteristic curve around the midbrain. On the left side, the posterior mesencephalic vein (4) communicates through a brachial vein (2) and the lateral anastomotic vein (1) with the petrosal vein (3). The petrosal vein is identified immediately above and slightly lateral to the internal auditory meatus which is penciled in. A large hemispheric vein is seen on the left side (h). The inferior vermian vein (arrowheads) in the midline communicates posteriorly with the torcula (T) and has an inferior hook (X) the copular point.

Superior (Galenic) Group[76]

The superior group of veins drains the superior aspect of the cerebellum and also the upper brainstem. The main route for drainage is into the great vein of Galen. The following veins are included in this group: the posterior mesencephalic veins, the precentral cerebellar vein, and the superior vermian vein.

Posterior Mesencephalic Veins

The posterior mesencephalic veins originate on the cerebral peduncle and course around the brainstem to drain into the great vein of Galen (Figs. 4-30, 4-31, 4-32). The description "posterior" is derived from the direction of blood flow. The vein receives blood from the mesencephalon and upper pons. Its course is identical to that of the basal vein of Rosenthal (and may on

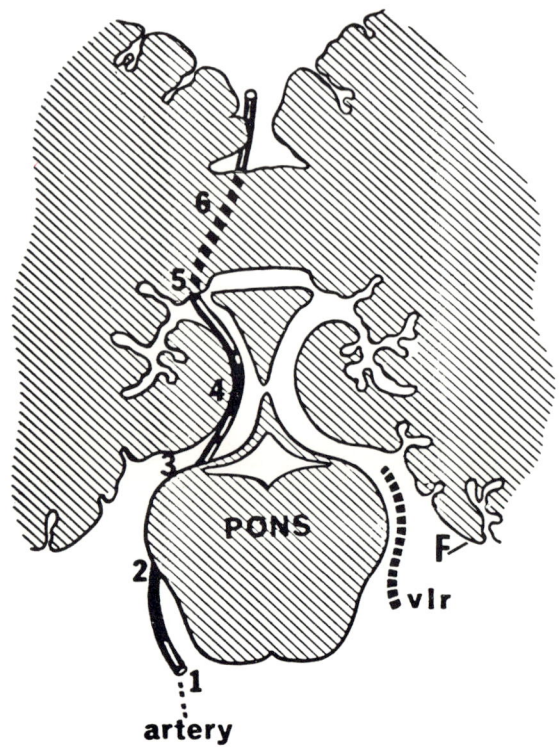

Fig. 4-33. Line diagram of the vein of the lateral recess of the fourth ventricle. The vein (vlr) lies in the posterolateral fissure and is bordered medially by the lower pons and laterally by the flocculus (F). On the right side (reader's left), the posterior inferior cerebellar artery is numbered as in Fig. 4-15.

occasions replace it), though it lies at a more caudal level and does not extend as far anteriorly as the basal vein of Rosenthal. The posterior mesencephalic vein extends posteriorly, superiorly, and medially.*

The posterior mesencephalic vein can communicate through a lateral mesencephalic vein with the brachial vein and subsequently communicate with the petrosal vein (Figs. 4-30, 4-31, 4-32). The lateral mesencephalic vein can also communicate with the basal vein of Rosenthal. When prominent, the

*There are eight vessels (four arteries and four veins) surrounding the midbrain which have, accordingly, similar configurations on angiography. The four arteries are the two posterior cerebral and the two superior cerebellar arteries; the four veins are the two basal veins of Rosenthal and the two posterior mesencephalic veins. All these structures lie completely or partly in the ambient cistern. While the four arteries are always present, on occasion, prominent basal veins of Rosenthal can substitute for absent posterior mesencephalic veins, and vice versa.

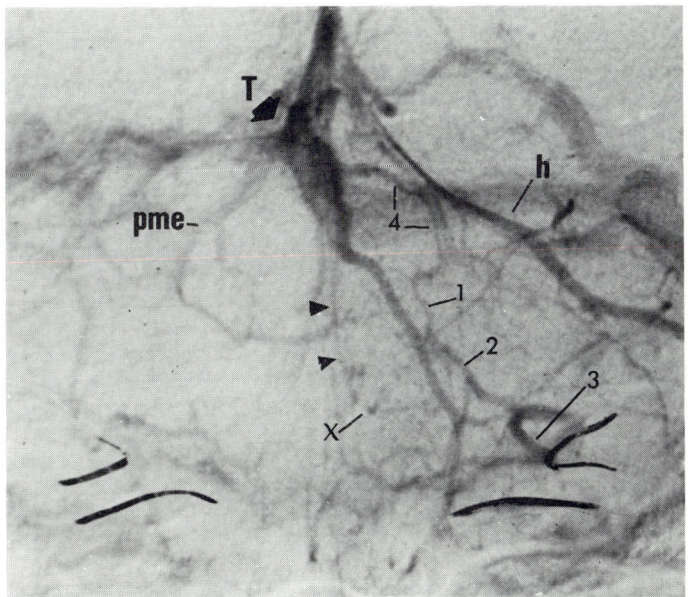

Fig. 4-34. Vertebral angiogram, venous phase, frontal projection. Two inferior vermian veins (i) lie parallel to each other in the inferior vermian sulcus. The vein of the lateral recess of the fourth ventricle (vlr) lies medial to the petrosal vein (p) and curves inferolaterally. Hemispheric veins (h) have arcuate courses as they lie on the surface of the cerebellar hemispheres.

lateral mesencephalic vein is called the lateral anastomotic mesencephalic vein and forms a communication between the supratentorial and infratentorial venous compartments.[83] The lateral mesencephalic vein is recognized by its vertical configuration parallel to the pontine vein and the inferior limb of the precentral cerebellar vein on the lateral projection (Fig. 4-30). In the semiaxial projection of an angiogram, it usually extends obliquely downward and laterally to the region of the internal auditory meatus.[76] The position and configuration in the semiaxial projection, however, may be variable.

Precentral Cerebellar Vein

The precentral cerebellar vein orignates in the depths of a fissure between the central lobule of the cerebellum and the roof of the lower aqueduct and upper fourth ventricle (Figs. 4-30, 4-36).[84] The vein originates from two brachial tributaries and runs initially superiorly in front of the central lobule of the cerebellum. This segment of the vein is usually parallel to both the lateral mesencephalic vein and the pontine vein. As the precentral cerebellar vein leaves the precentral fissure, it turns backward immediately behind the inferior

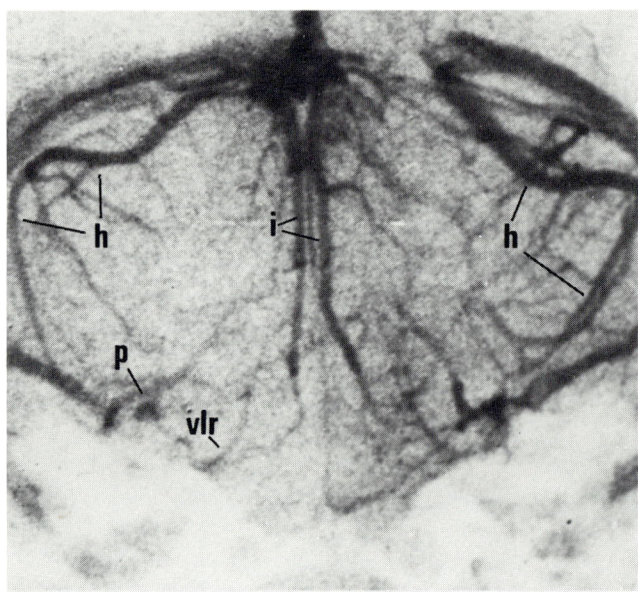

Fig. 4-35. Vertebral angiogram, venous phase, frontal projection. An isolated vermian vein (i) curves inferiorly to communicate with the petrosal vein (p) forming a venous link between it and the torcula (T). The vein of the lateral recess (vlr) is faintly seen running inferolaterally from the region of the lateral recess of the fourth ventricle. Anterior to the pons, transverse pontine veins (tp) separate the pons from the pontine cistern and clivus (C).

colliculi to form a characteristic knee, called the colliculo-central angle. The most anterior point of this angle is called the colliculo-central point (Figs. 4-30, 4-36). Deformities and displacements of the colliculo-central point correlate with changes in the upper part of the fourth ventricle and the aqueduct. Above the colliculo-central point, the precentral cerebellar vein runs within the quadrigeminal cistern to empty either into the superior vermian vein or directly into the great vein of Galen. The precentral cerebellar vein is easily recognized on the lateral projection, but there is difficulty in recognizing the vein in the semiaxial projection due to overlap by the inferior vermian veins.*

*A useful measurement for the position of the colliculo-central point is to drop a line perpendicular to Twining's line (tuberculum sella-torcula). The perpendicular should, on the average, bisect Twining's line (44%–55%).[84] Huang et al. also found that the distance between the most posterior and inferior portion of the ponto-mesencephalic vein in the interpeduncular fossa and the colliculo-central point measured between 18 and 23 mm with an average of 21 mm.[77] The distance between the anterior aspect of the belly of the pons (outlined by the ponto-mesencephalic vein) and the colliculo-central point measured between 29 and 36 mm with a mean of 32 mm. The minimum distance between the clivus and the colliculo-central point measured between 36 and 43 mm with a mean of 39 mm.[84]

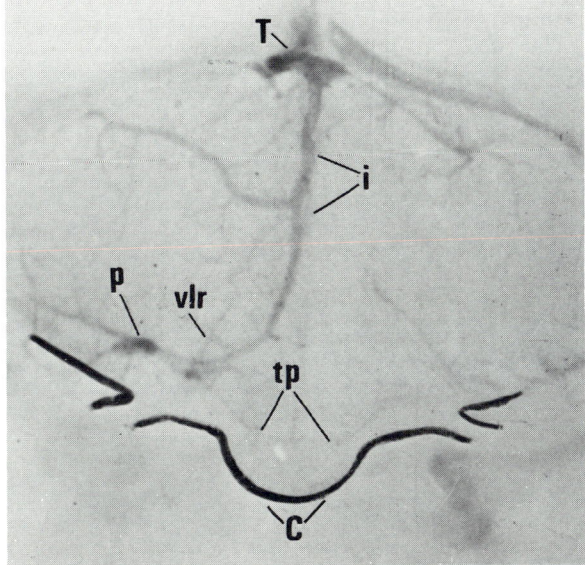

Fig. 4-36. An angiotomogram (same case as 4-30). Angiotomography demonstrates the midline precentral cerebellar vein (p) with the colliculo-central point (X) and the inferior vermian vein (arrowheads).

Superior Vermian Vein

The superior vermian vein drains the superior vermis and adjacent portions of the hemisphere (Figs. 4-30, 4-31, 4-37).[76] The vein reaches the anterosuperior margin of the cerebellum, dips down into the precentral cerebellar fissure, and then ascends to enter the great vein of Galen. Frequently, a single vein is not present. Instead, there are two separate veins on either side of the midline. On the lateral projection, the superior vermian vein and its tributaries are easily seen. The distance between the superior vermian vein and the straight sinus represents the superior cerebellar cistern. Obliteration of this cistern is an indirect sign of a cerebellar vermian mass. The superior vermian vein is frequently difficult to define in the semiaxial projection due to overlap by the inferior vermian veins.

Posterior (Tentorial) Group

Included in the posterior (tentorial) group are the inferior vermian and inferior hemispheric veins.

Inferior Vermian Vein

The major vein draining the inferior vermis is the inferior vermian vein (Figs. 4-30, 4-31, 4-32, 4-34, 4-35, 4-36).[26] It is formed by union of superior and inferior retrotonsillar tributaries immediately anterior to the copula pyramidal lobe of the cerebellum. As it hooks under the pyramidal lobe, it makes a characteristic loop that can be easily recognized on the lateral angiogram (Figs. 4-30, 4-31). The most anterior point of the curve of the pyramidal loop is called the copular point.* The vein then extends posterosuperiorly.

Since the inferior vermian vein outlines the inferior vermis which lies at a greater depth than the cerebellar hemisphere, on a lateral angiogram the vein is separated from the occipital squamosa. The hemispheric veins, on the other hand, lie adjacent to the squamosa.

Usually two inferior vermian veins are present parallel to each other in the inferior vermian sulcus.

Angiotomography helps to distinguish the midline veins, the inferior vermian and precentral veins, from more laterally situated veins (Fig. 4-36).

SUPRATENTORIAL VEINS

Since vertebral angiography opacifies supratentorial structures supplied by the posterior cerebral artery and its branches, supratentorial veins draining the mesencephalon, posterior portion of the diencephalon, the lateral ventricle, the occipital lobe, the posterior temporal lobe, and the posterior parietal lobe can be visualized.[85]

Basal Vein of Rosenthal

The course of the basal vein of Rosenthal is parallel to that of the posterior mesencephalic vein and lies immediately above it. The vein commences in the interpeduncular fossa and then courses posteriorly and superiorly in the crural and ambient cisterns to end in the great vein of Galen. Opacification of the vein after vertebral angiography is variable, whereas it is almost always visualized after carotid angiography. Generally, only the posterior segment of the vein is opacified after vertebral angiography. If the posterior segment is congenitally absent, however, the anterior segment drains into the petrosal vein via the lateral anastomotic mesencephalic vein.[83]

---

*Huang and associates have related the copular point to the midpoint of a line joining the torcula and the anterior lip of the foramen magnum.[26] They found that the copular point fell within a circle of 6 mm radius with its center 4 mm behind and below the midpoint.

Thalamic Veins

Guidicelli and Salamon described four thalamic veins on each side: the superior, anterior, inferior, and posterior thalamic veins.[86] The superior vein drains the posterior and superior aspect of the thalamus and runs below and parallel to the internal cerebral vein to drain into the terminal portion of the internal cerebral vein, or into the basal vein of Rosenthal. The anterior thalamic vein drains the anterior aspect of the thalamus and courses anterosuperiorly to enter into the internal cerebral vein at the foramen of Monro. According to Takahashi and Okudera, the anterior and superior thalamic veins are visualized in the majority of good-quality vertebral angiograms.[87] The inferior and posterior thalamic veins, which drain into the basal vein of Rosenthal, are seen in the minority of cases.

Choroid Plexus and Superior Choroidal Veins

The choroid plexus in the floor of the body of the lateral ventricle is seen in 84 percent of lateral angiograms as a faint blush in the late arterial through to the venous phase of the vertebral angiogram.[87] The superior choroidal vein is seen as interrupted lines or band-like densities within the choroidal blush. The blush on a semiaxial projection appears as an arcuate band-like density convex superiorly.

Internal Cerebral Vein

Takahashi and Okudera have identified the internal cerebral vein in 97 percent of vertebral angiograms.[87]

Occipital Veins

Veins draining the occipital lobe, posterior parietal, and posterior temporal lobes drain into the sagittal and lateral sinuses. Vein over the cuneus drain into the straight sinus or vein of Galen.

Variations

Since the cerebral veins develop from embryologically derived venous plexuses, variations are frequent.[76]

The ponto-mesencephalic vein, instead of draining inferiorly to the petrosal vein, may drain into the superior (Galenic) group of veins by anterior communication with the basal vein of Rosenthal and posterior mesencephalic vein.[77,88] The ponto-mesencephalic vein may also drain directly into the cavernous sinus, the basilar plexus, or the inferior petrosal sinus.[77] On occa-

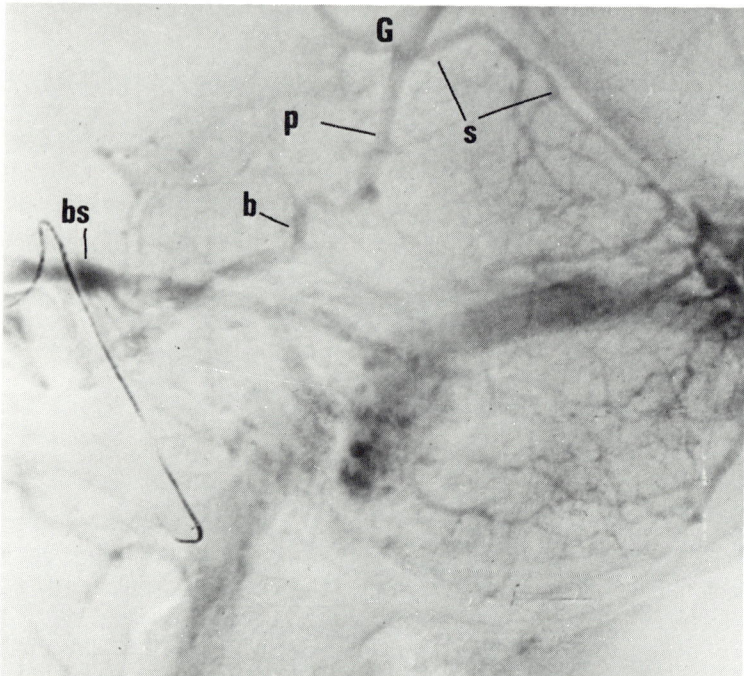

Fig. 4-37. Left vertebral angiogram, venous phase, lateral projection: same case as Fig. 4-38. The precentral cerebellar vein (p) communicates through a brachial vein (b) with the superior petrosal sinus which in turn communicates with the basal venous plexus (bs). A large supraculminate vein (s) unites with the precentral cerebellar vein. Together the two veins enter the great vein of Galen (G). Posteriorly, the supraculminate vein descends as the superior vermian vein over the declive of the cerebellum. The superior vermis can be easily defined.

sions, the ponto-mesencephalic vein may not lie in the midline, but on the anterolateral aspect of the pons.[77] Instead of a single vein, two anterior ponto-mesencephalic veins may be present side by side.[78] Occasionally, the ponto-mesencephalic veins may be seen on carotid angiography.[78]

When a lateral anastomotic mesencephalic vein is present, the posterior segment of the basal vein of Rosenthal is usually absent, since the basal vein of Rosenthal will then drain into the petrosal vein.[83]

The two brachial tributaries of the precentral cerebellar vein may remain separate, in which case two separate venous trunks may be seen. The precentral cerebellar vein is not present in all patients. In such cases, the brachial veins drain anteriorly into the petrosal veins. If the precentral cerebellar vein lies to one side of the midline, it lies more anteriorly than the normal precentral cerebellar vein and does not show the typical angulation.[84] The precentral

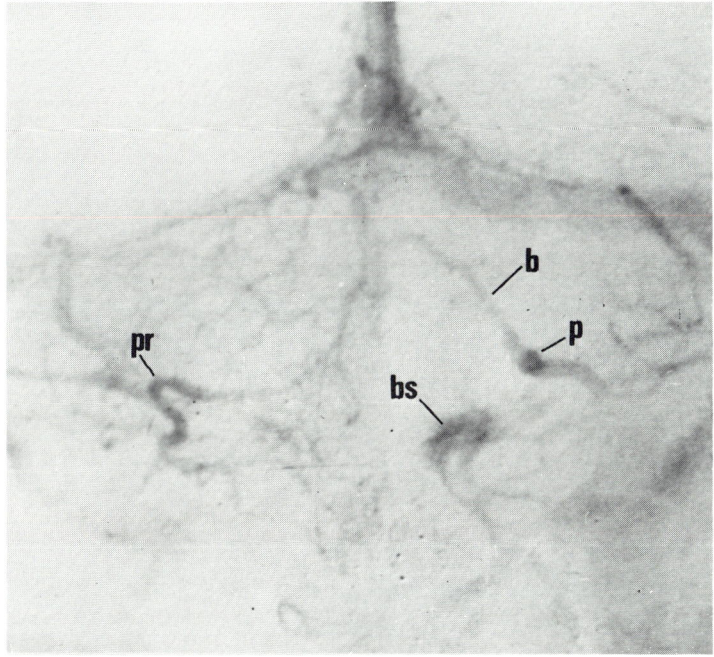

Fig. 4-38. Frontal projection. The brachial vein (b) drains into the petrosal vein (p) on the left side. The petrosal vein communicates with the basal venous plexus (bs). The right petrosal vein (pr) is also indicated.

cerebellar vein may form a communication between the great vein of Galen and the petrosal vein (Figs. 4-37, 4-38).

The inferior vermian vein may not run in the inferior vermian sulcus for the entire course but may leave the sulcus and run upward on the inferior surface of the cerebellar hemisphere to empty into the transverse sinus.[26]

REFERENCES

1. Gray H: Gray's Anatomy (ed 28) Philadelphia, Lea & Febiger, 1966
2. Brain R: Order and disorder in the cerebral circulation. Lancet 2:857, 1957
3. Stopford JSB: The arteries of the pons and medulla oblongata. J Anat Physiol 50:131, 1916
4. Williams DJ: The origin of the posterior cerebral artery. Brain 59:175, 1936
5. Schechter MM: The occipital-vertebral anastomosis. J Neurosurg 21:758, 1964
6. Nierling DA, Wollschlaeger PB, Wollschlaeger G: Ascending pharyngeal-vertebral anastomosis. Am J Roentgenol 98:599, 1966
7. Pakula H, Szapiro J: Anatomical studies of the collateral blood supply to the brain and upper extremity. J Neurosurg 32:171, 1970
8. Stehbens WE: Pathology of the Cerebral Vessels. St. Louis, Mosby, 1972

9. Schechter MM, Zingesser LH: The spinal arteries. Acta Radiol [Diagn](Stockh) 5:1124, 1966
10. Billewicz O, Heldt N: The visualization of the anterior spinal artery and its blood-stream direction during brachial vertebral angiography. Neuroradiology 2:46, 1971
11. Gabrielsen TP, Seeger JF, Crane JD: Veins of the upper cervical spinal cord in vertebral angiography. Acta Radiol [Diagn] (Stockh) 13:801, 1972
12. Marc JA, Schechter MM: Radiological diagnosis of mass lesions within and adjacent to the foramen magnum. Radiology 114:351, 1975
13. Krayenbühl HA, Yaşargil MG: Cerebral Angiography (ed 2). Philadelphia, Lippincott, 1968
14. Huang, YP, Wolf BS: Angiographic features of fourth ventricle tumors with special reference to the posterior inferior cerebellar artery. Am J Roentgenol 197:543, 1969
15. Greitz T, Sjögren SE: The posterior inferior cerebellar artery. Acta Radiol [Diagn] (Stockh) 1:284, 1963
16. Margolis MT, Newton TH: Borderlands of the normal and abnormal posterior inferior cerebellar artery. Acta Radiol [Diagn] (Stockh) 13:163, 1972
17. Wolf BS, Newman CM, Khilnani MT: The posterior inferior artery on vertebral angiography. Am J Roentgenol 87:322, 1962
18. Megret M: A landmark for the choroidal arteries of the fourth ventricle—branches of the posterior inferior cerebellar artery. Neuroradiology 5:85, 1973
19. Peeters FL: Angiography of the vertebral artery in the diagnosis of tumours of the pons cerebelli. A preliminary report. Radiol Clin Biol 37:89, 1968
20. Peeters FL: The vertebral angiogram in patients with tumours in or near the midline. Neuroradiology 5:53, 1973
21. Belloni G, duBoulay G: The choroidal point and copular point. Br J Radiol 47:261, 1974
22. Sahlstedt H: Writing in Lysholm's Das Ventriculogram, I. Teil. Acta Radiol (Suppl) (Stockh) 24, 1935
23. Twining EW: Radiology of the third and fourth ventricle, part 2. Br J Radiol 12:569, 1939
24. Takahashi M, Okudera T, Fukui M, Kitamura K: The choroidal and nodular branches of the posterior inferior cerebellar artery. Their value in the diagnosis of medulloblastomas. Radiology 103:347, 1972
25. Leman P, Cohadon F, Leifer C: Description des Trajets Normaux des Artères de la Fosse Postérieure. Ann Radiol 10:781, 1967
26. Huang YP, Wolf BS, Okudera T: Angiographic anatomy of the inferior vermian vein of the cerebellum. Acta Radiol [Diagn] (Stockh) 9:327, 1969
27. Margolis MT, Newton TH: The posterior inferior cerebellar artery, in Newton TH, Potts DG (eds): Radiology of the Skull and Brain, vol 2, book 2. St. Louis, Mosby, 1974, p 1710
28. Taveras JM, Wood EH: Diagnostic Neuroradiology. Baltimore, Williams & Wilkins, 1964
29. Radner S: Vertebral angiography by catheterization. A new method employed in 221 cases. Acta Radiol (Suppl) (Stockh) 87, 1951
30. Lie TA: Congenital Anomalies of the Carotid Arteries. Amsterdam, Excerpta Medica Foundation, 1968
31. Ouchi H, OHara I: Extracranial abnormalities of the vertebral artery detected by selective arteriography. J Cardiovasc Surg (Torino) 9:250, 1968
32. Conforti P, Armenise B, Galligioni F: Anomalous carotid-vertebral anastomosis: primitive cervical segmental artery. Neurochirurgia (Stuttg) 9:99, 1966
33. Hutchinson NA, Miller JDR: Persistent proatlantal artery. J Neurol Neurosurg Psychiatry 33:524, 1970
34. Flynn RE: External carotid origin of the dominant vertebral artery. J Neurosurg 29:300, 1968
35. Mizukami M, Tomita T, Mine T, Mihara H: Bypass anomaly of the vertebral artery associated with cerebral aneurysm and arteriovenous malformation. J Neurosurg 37:204, 1972

36. Handa H, Handa J, Koyama T: Agenesis of the corpus callosum associated with multiple anomalies of the cerebral arteries: report of a case and review of the literature. Brain Nerve (Tokyo) 20:317, 1968
37. Berry RJA, Anderson JJ: A case of Nonunion of the Vertebrales with consequent abnormal Origin of the Basilaris. Anat Anz 35:54, 1909
38. McCullough AW: Some anomalies of the cerebral arterial circle (of Willis) and related vessels. Anat Rec 143:537, 1962
39. McMinn RMH: A case of non-union of the vertebral arteries. Anat Rec 116:283, 1953
40. Gillilan LA: The correlation of the blood supply to the human brain stem with clinical brain stem lesions. J Neuropathol Exp Neurol 23:78, 1964
41. Takahashi M, Wilson G, Hanafee W: The anterior inferior cerebellar artery: its radiographic anatomy and significance in the diagnosis of extra-axial tumors of the posterior fossa. Radiology 90:281, 1968
42. Stephens RB, Stilwell DL: Arteries and Veins of the Human Brain. Springfield, Charles C Thomas, 1969
43. Sugarman DA: Observations on the vertebral and basilar arteries and their branches in man, with special reference to the lateral parolivary fossa. M J Australia 2:420, 1950
44. Haverling M: The tortuous basilar artery. Acta Radiol [Diagn] (Stockh) 15:241, 1975
45. Atkinson WJ: The anterior inferior cerebellar artery: its variations, pontine distribution, and significance in surgery of cerebello-pontine angle tumours. J Neurol Neurosurg Psychiatry 12:137, 1949
46. Gerald B, Wolpert SM, Haimovici H: The angiographic anatomy of the anterior inferior cerebellar artery. Am J Roentgenol 118:617, 1973
47. Mazzoni A: Internal auditory canal arterial relations at the porus acusticus. Ann Otolaryngol 78:797, 1969
48. Sunderland S: The arterial relations of the internal auditory meatus. Brain 68:23, 1945
49. Smaltino F, Bernini FP, Elefante R: Normal and pathological findings of the angiographic examination of the internal auditory artery. Neuroradiology 2:216, 1971
50. Gabrielsen TO, Amundsen P: The pontine arteries in vertebral angiography. Am J Roentgenol 106:296, 1969a
51. Walker EA, Jr: The vertebro-basilar arterial system and internal auditory angiography. Laryngoscope 75:369, 1965
52. Mani RL, Newton TH, Glickman MG: The superior cerebellar artery: an anatomic roentgenographic correlation. Radiology 91:1102, 1968
53. Huang YP, Wolf BS, Antin SP, Okudera T, Kim IH: Angiographic features of aqueductal stenosis. Am J Roentgenol 104:90, 1968b
54. Margolis MT, Newton TH, Hoyt, WF: Cortical branches of the posterior cerebral artery. Anatomic-radiologic correlation. Neuroradiology 2:127, 1971
55. Galloway JR, Greitz T, Sjögren SE: Vertebral angiography in the diagnosis of ventricular dilatation. Acta Radiol [Diagn] (Stockh) 2:321, 1964
56. Westberg G: Arteries of the basal ganglia. Acta Radiol [Diagn] (Stockh) 5:581, 1966
57. Hara K, Fujino Y: The thalamoperforate artery. Acta Radiol [Diagn] (Stockh) 5:192, 1966
58. Löfgren FO: Vertebral angiography in the diagnosis of tumours in the pineal region. Acta Radiol 50:108, 1958
59. Galloway JR, Greitz T: The medial and lateral choroid arteries. An anatomic and roentgenographic study. Acta Radiol [Diagn] (Stockh) 53:353, 1960
60. Takahashi M, Tamakawa Y, Kishikawa T, Kowaoa M: Fenestration of the basilar artery. Report of three cases and review of the literature. Radiology 109:79, 1973
61. Gillilan LA: Significant superficial anastomoses in the arterial blood supply to the human brain. J Comp Neurol 112:55, 1959
62. Alpers BJ, Berry RG, Paddison RM: Anatomical studies of the Circle of Willis in normal brain. Arch Neurol Psychiatr 81:409, 1959

63. Newton TH: The anterior and posterior meningeal branches of the vertebral artery. Radiology 91:271, 1968
64. Salamon GM, Combalbert A, Raybaud C, Gonzalez J: An angiographic study of meningiomas of the posterior fossa. J Neurosurg 35:731, 1971
65. Dilenge D, David M: La branche méningée de l'artère vertebrale. Neurochirurgia (Stuttg) 8:121, 1965
66. Hawkins TD, Melcher: A meningeal artery in the falx cerebelli. Clin Radiol 17:377, 1966
67. Djindjian R, Théron J: Unpublished data, 1974
68. Greitz T, Laurén T: Anterior meningeal branch of the vertebral artery. Acta Radiol [Diagn] (Stockh) 7:219, 1968
69. Schnürer LB, Stattin S: Vascular supply of intracranial dura from internal carotid artery with special reference to its angiographic significance. Acta Radiol [Diagn] (Stockh) 1:441, 1963
70. McConnell EM: The arterial blood supply of the human hypophysis cerebri. Anat Rec 115:175, 1953
71. Parkinson D: Collateral circulation of cavernous carotid artery: anatomy. Can J Surg 7:251, 1964
72. Théron J, Lasjaunias P: Participation of the external and internal carotid arteries in the vascular supply of cerebellopontine angle tumours. Thirteenth Annual Meeting of American Society of Neuroradiology, Vancouver, B.C., 1975
73. Théron J, Djindjian R: Cervicovertebral phlebography using catheterization. A preliminary report. Radiology 108:325, 1973
74. Backmund H, Grusche A, Schmidt-Vanderheyden W: Venous pattern in normal lateral serial angiograms of the carotid artery. Neuroradiology 3:20, 1971
75. Dilenge D, Perey B: An angiographic study of the venous system. Radiology 108:333, 1973
76. Huang YP, Wolf BS: The veins of the posterior fossa—superior or galenic draining group. Am J Roentgenol 95:808, 1965
77. Huang YP, Wolf BS, Antin SP, Okudera T: The veins of the posterior fossa—anterior or petrosal draining group. Am J Roentgenol 104:36, 1968a
78. Gabrielsen TO, Amundsen P: The pontomesencephalic veins. A roentgenographic study. Radiology 92:889, 1969b
79. Huang YP, Wolf BS: The vein of the lateral recess of the fourth ventricle and its tributaries. Roentgen appearance and anatomic relationships. Am J Roentgenol 101:1, 1967
80. Braun JP, Tournade A: The veins of the lateral recess of the 4th ventricle. Neuroradiology 9:9, 1974
81. Takahashi M, Wilson G, Hanafee W: The significance of the petrosal vein in the diagnosis of cerebellopontine angle tumors. Radiology 89:834, 1967
82. Bull J, Kozlowski P: The angiographic pattern of the petrosal veins in the normal and pathological. Neuroradiology 1:20, 1970
83. Wolf BS, Huang YP, Newman CM: The lateral anastomotic mesencephalic vein and other variations in drainage of the basal cerebral vein. Am J Roentgenol 89:411, 1963
84. Huang YP, Wolf BS: Precentral cerebellar vein in angiography. Acta Radiol [Diagn] (Stockh) 5:250, 1966
85. Takahashi M: Atlas of Vertebral Angiography. Tokyo, Igaku Shoin Ltd, 1974
86. Guidicelli G, Salamon G: The veins of the thalamus. Neuroradiology 1:92, 1970
87. Takahashi M, Okudera T: The choroid plexus and the choroid vein of the lateral ventricle. Their angiographic appearance and clinical significance. Radiology 103:113, 1972
88. Bradac GB: The ponto-mesencephalic veins (Radio-anatomical study). Neuroradiology 1:52, 1970

5
Prepontine and Cerebellopontine Angle Tumors
(Plate III*)

Acoustic neurinomas, meningiomas, epidermoids, and chordomas are the most common tumors found in the pontine and cerebellopontine angle cisterns. Gliomas and ependymomas can also rarely present as extra-axial masses in the cerebellopontine angle. The gliomas arise as exophytic masses originating from pontine gliomas. The ependymomas grow out of the fourth ventricle and into the cerebellopontine angle. Other rare lesions presenting as tumors of the angle include arachnoid cysts, metastatic tumors to the petrous bone, glomus jugulare tumors, choroid plexus papillomas, aneurysms of the basilar artery, anterior inferior cerebellar artery, and vertebral artery, and neurinomas of the fifth, seventh, tenth, and twelfth cranial nerves.[1,2] Marked dilatation of the anterior third ventricle can also present as a prepontine tumor.[3]

Rarely, mucoceles of the sphenoid sinus, optic nerve gliomas, and pituitary adenomas can also present as prepontine tumors.[4] In children, embryonal rhabdomyosarcomas can originate from the middle ear, erode through the petrous bone, and present as extra-axial brainstem tumors.[5,6] Craniopharyngiomas can also present as prepontine tumors when the tumors grow down the clivus.

Acoustic neurinomas are the most frequent tumors of the cerebellopontine angle; they constitute over 90 percent of the neoplasms in this area.[7] Though usually single, they may be bilateral, in which case they are usually associated with the neurofibromatosis of van Recklinghausen's disease.[8] There is also a

*See color plate, page 33.

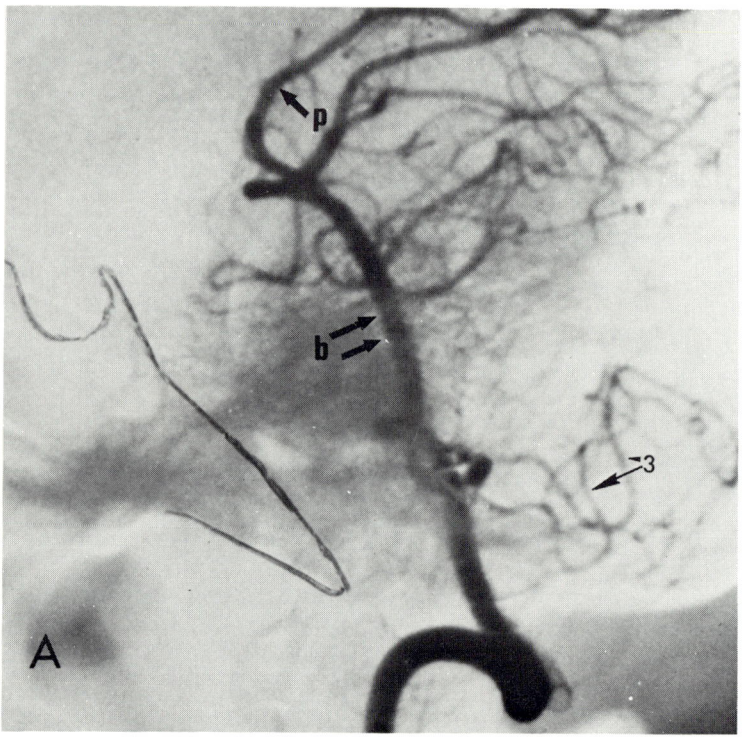

relatively high incidence of meningiomas in the presence of acoustic neurinomas.[9]

Meningiomas in the posterior fossa contribute between 6.0 and 13.4 percent of all intracranial meningiomas. They may occur on the clivus, on the posterior surface of the petrous bone, at the edge of the foramen magnum, on the edge of the tentorium, or over the cerebellar convexity. According to Castellano and Ruggiero, they most often occur on the posterior surface of the petrous bone.[10]

Epidermoids are congenital tumors which can occur in the cerebellopontine angle. They are called primary cholesteatomas to distinguish them from cholesteatomas secondary to infections of the middle ear.

Chordomas occurring in the skull are very rare tumors. They are regionally invasive, but otherwise benign, and are extradural in location. Typically, they cause marked bone destruction with considerable soft-tissue calcification.[11, 12] Macroscopically and radiologically, chondromas of the skull base can appear identical to chordomas.[13]

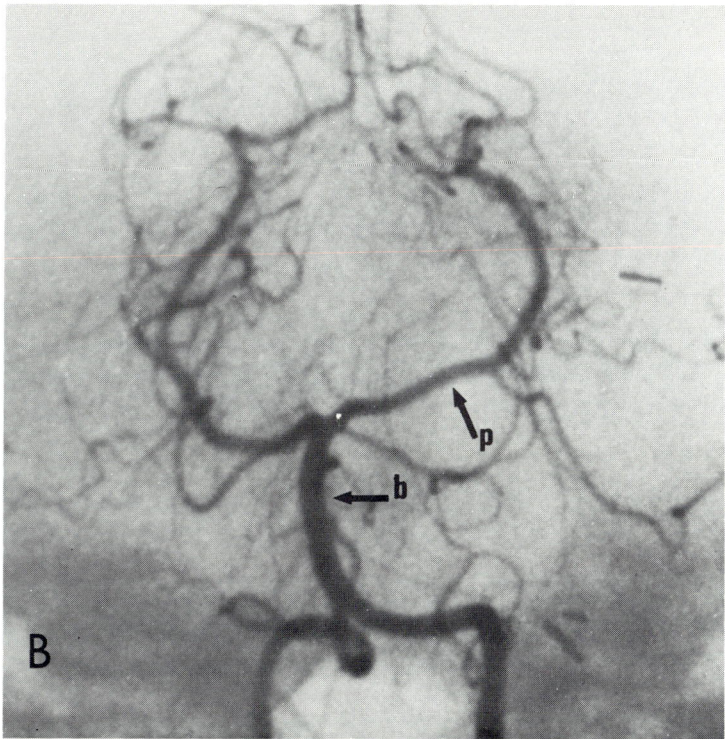

Fig. 5-1A,B. Prepontine meningioma. Left vertebral angiogram, arterial phase, lateral and frontal projections. The basilar artery (b) is displaced backward and to the right. The tumor has extended into the left cerebellopontine angle causing brainstem rotation. Both posterior medullary segments (3) of PICA are opacified with the left segment lying posterior to the right. The left posterior cerebral artery (p) is elevated.

PREPONTINE TUMORS

The angiographic hallmark of a prepontine mass is posterior displacement of the basilar artery.[4,14,15] The artery is displaced in an arc, anteriorly concave, and may also be laterally displaced if the mass extends into the cerebellopontine angle (Figs. 5-1A,B, 5-2A,B, also see 5-8).[16] Associated with the displacement of the basilar artery is posterior displacement of the ponto-mesencephalic vein, if the mass is present behind the dorsum sellae (Fig. 5-3A,B).[17] In cases of clival chordomas, the petrocavernous part of the internal carotid artery may be displaced anteriorly (Fig. 5-8).

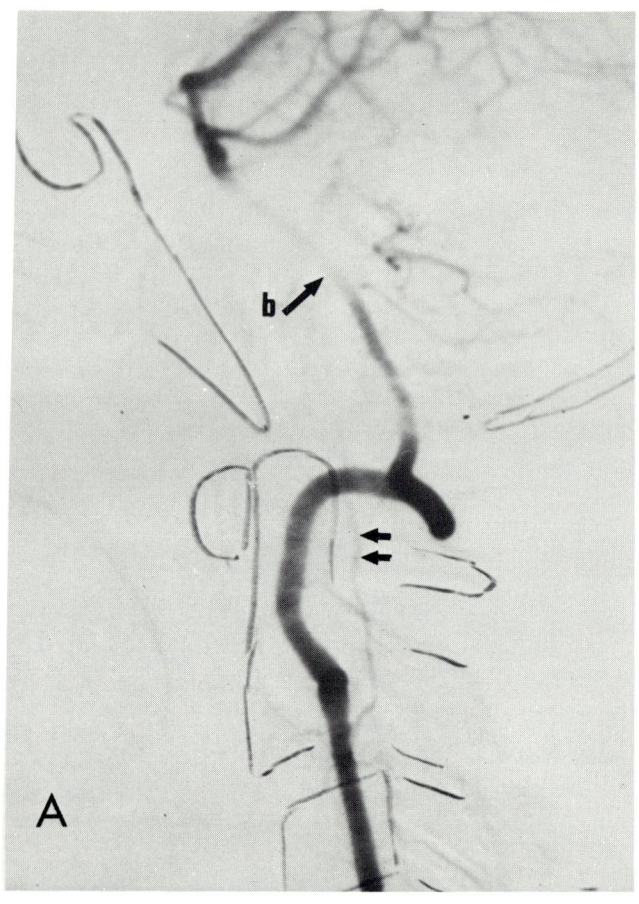

Hypertrophied dorsal clival arteries have been described with clival meningiomas (Fig. 5-6A,B), fifth nerve neurinomas, chordomas, and acoustic neurinomas.[18-21] An irregular network of pathological vessels was described in one of Radner's four cases of clival meningioma.[22] More frequently the tumor appears as a uniformly homogeneous stain (Fig. 5-7). Angiographic studies of patients with chondromas, however, stress the avascularity of the lesions.[23] When tumors originate adjacent to the anterior rim of the foramen magnum, the anterior meningeal branch of the vertebral artery may be enlarged (Fig. 5-2A,B). This has been described with meningiomas, glomus jugulare tumors, metastatic tumors to the lower clivus, plasmocytomas, chordomas and schwannomas.[24-27] A clival meningioma may also derive its blood supply

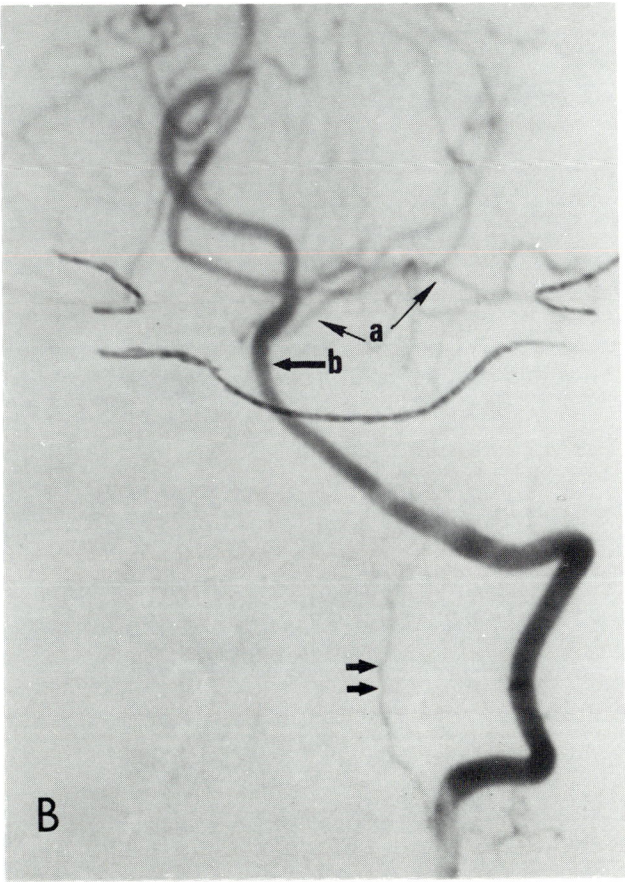

Fig. 5-2A,B. Prepontine meningioma. Left vertebral angiogram, arterial phase, lateral and frontal projections: same case as Figs. 5-3A,B, 5-4. The basilar artery (b) is displaced backward and to the right. The tumor is elevating the anterior inferior cerebellar artery (a). Note the hypertrophied anterior meningeal branch of the vertebral artery (paired arrows).

from meningeal branches of the ascending pharyngeal artery (Figs. 5-5A,B).[18] When a meningioma is yet more lateral and closer to the convexity, branches of the middle meningeal and occipital arteries are likely to supply it (see Figs. 8-24A,B).[18, 28]

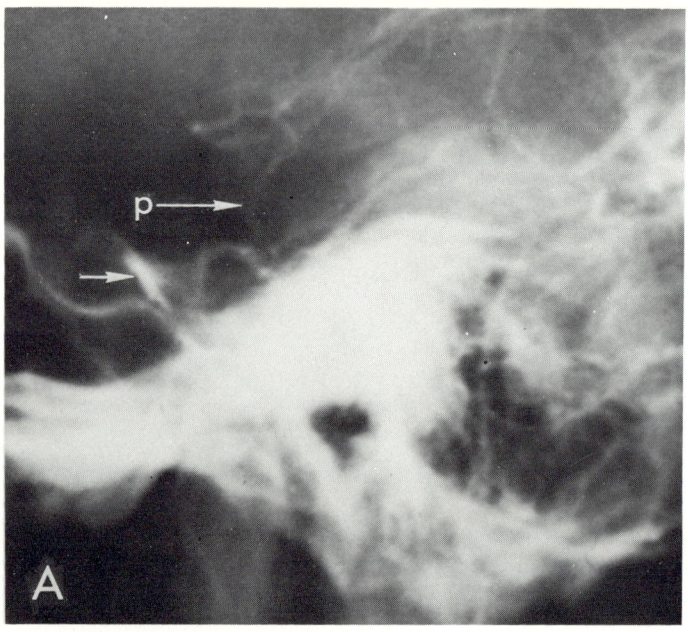

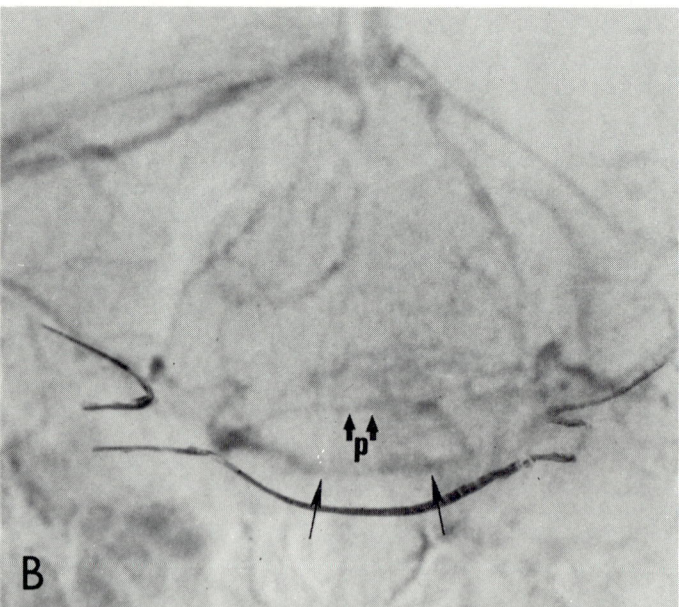

Fig. 5-3A,B. Venous phase, lateral and frontal projections. The ponto-mesencephalic vein (p) is displaced backward. The basal venous plexus (unlabeled arrow on lateral projection) adjacent to the dorsum sellae must not be confused with the ponto-mesencephalic vein. In the frontal projection, a posteriorly displaced transverse vein is seen extending laterally (two arrows). Fig. 5-3A is a non-subtracted film.

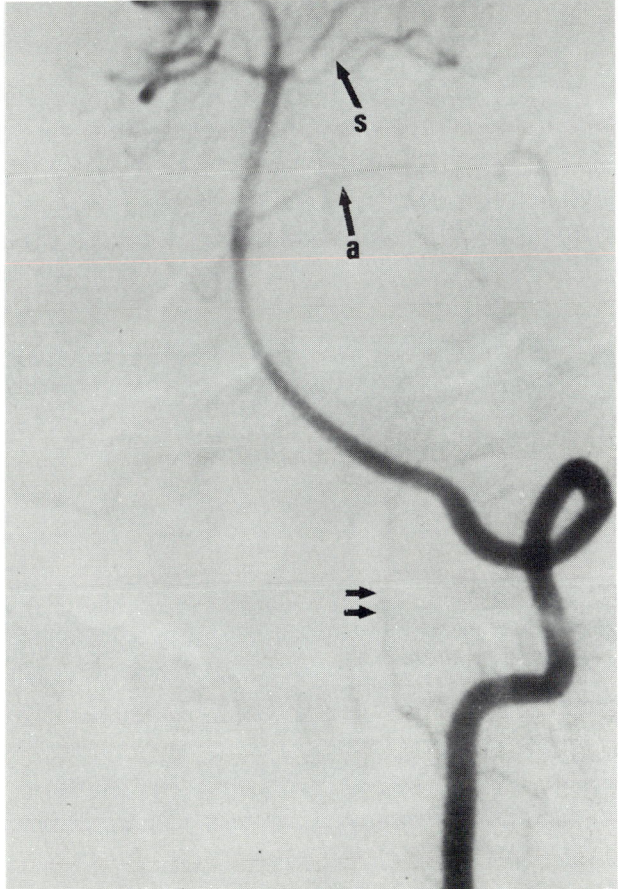

Fig. 5-4. Arterial phase, Caldwell projection. Note the elevation of the anterior inferior cerebellar artery (a) and the superior cerebellar artery (s) indicating a cerebellopontine angle tumor. The lower two arrows indicate the anterior meningeal branch of the vertebral artery.

CEREBELLOPONTINE ANGLE TUMORS

When the tumors originate in or extend into the cerebellopontine angle, the major vascular displacements involve the anterior inferior cerebellar artery and the petrosal vein. While the anterior inferior cerebellar artery is usually elevated, it may depressed (Figs. 5-4, 5-9, 5-19).[23,29,30] Since the anterior inferior cerebellar artery normally takes a downward course, downward depression is difficult to appreciate whereas elevation is easy.[31] In

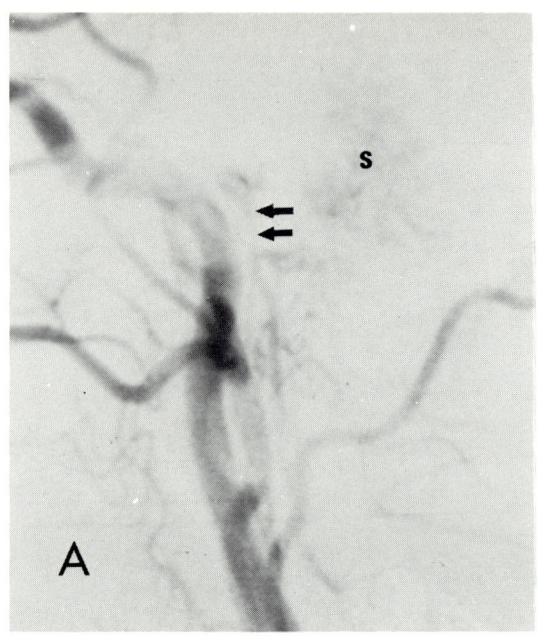

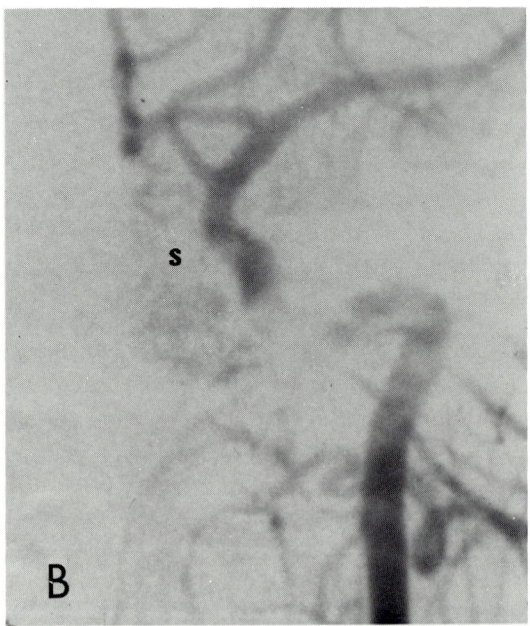

Fig. 5-5A,B. Clival meningioma. Left carotid angiogram, arterial phase, lateral and frontal projections. The ascending pharyngeal artery (double arrows) is hypertrophied and supplies the tumor which is visualized as a vascular stain (s).

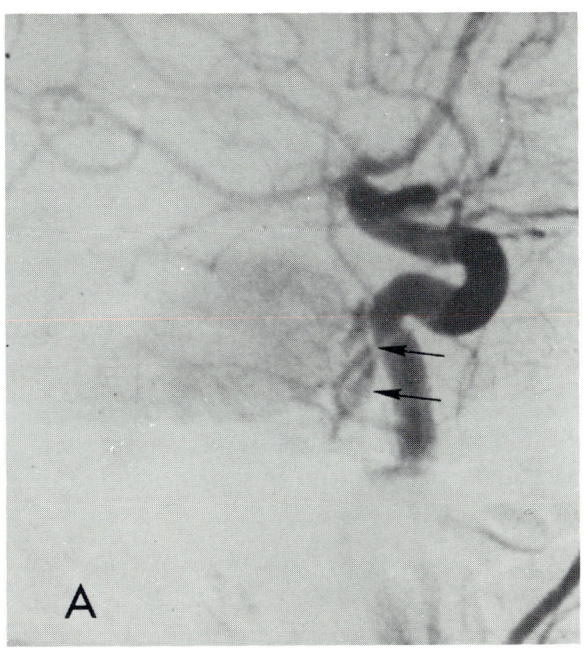

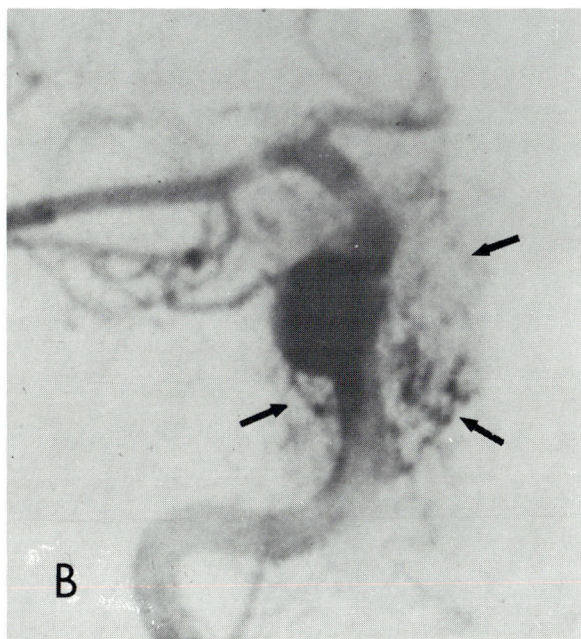

Fig. 5-6A,B. Clival meningioma. Left carotid angiogram, arterial phase, lateral and frontal projections: same case as Fig. 5-7. Note the hypertrophied dorsal clival artery (paired arrows) ending in a tumor stain. The tumor stain (arrows) is seen behind the petrocavernous segment of the internal carotid artery in the frontal projection.

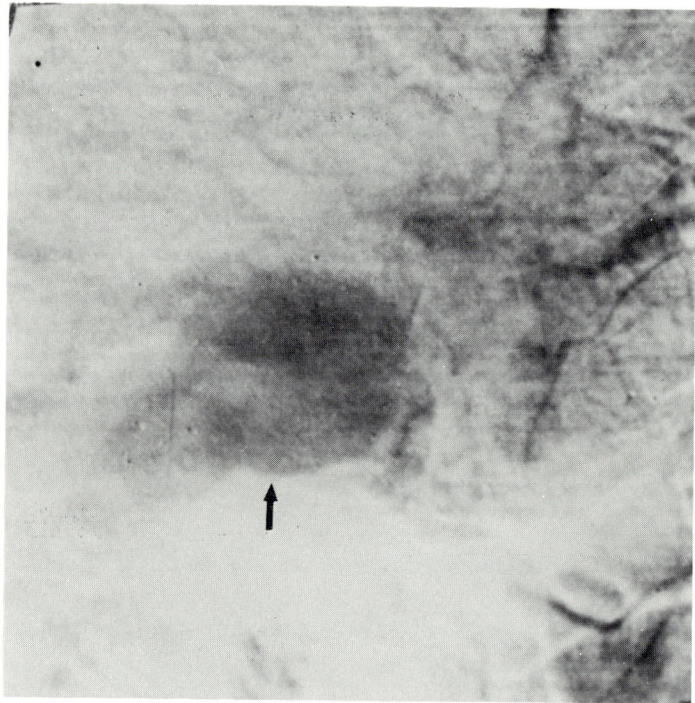

Fig. 5-7. Lateral projection. In the intermediate phase, a dense vascular tumor stain is seen behind the clivus (arrow).

addition to the more common tumors, chromophobe adenomas, craniopharyngiomas, chordomas, and trigeminal neurinomas may depress the anterior inferior cerebellar artery.

Stretching and displacement of the cerebellolabryinthine and internal auditory arteries were described by Smaltino and associates in cases of acoustic neurinomas.[32] The displacement depends on the direction of the growth of the tumor. A Caldwell projection is ideal for demonstrating the anterior inferior cerebellar artery (Figs. 4-22, 5-4, 5-10). On occasions, acoustic neurinomas may derive their blood supply exclusively from the middle meningeal artery through its supply to the dura mater adjacent to the trigeminal nerve, as well as from the dorsal clival artery.[21] (See Chapter 9.)

The petrosal vein is usually elevated, though it may be compressed and obliterated by the angle tumor (Figs. 5-11, 5-12, 5-13).[17,33-36] Veins draining into the petrosal vein, such as the lateral anastomotic mesencephalic vein, the vein of the lateral recess of the fourth ventricle, transverse pontine, and hemispheric veins may be similarly displaced.[36] Abnormal, enlarged veins

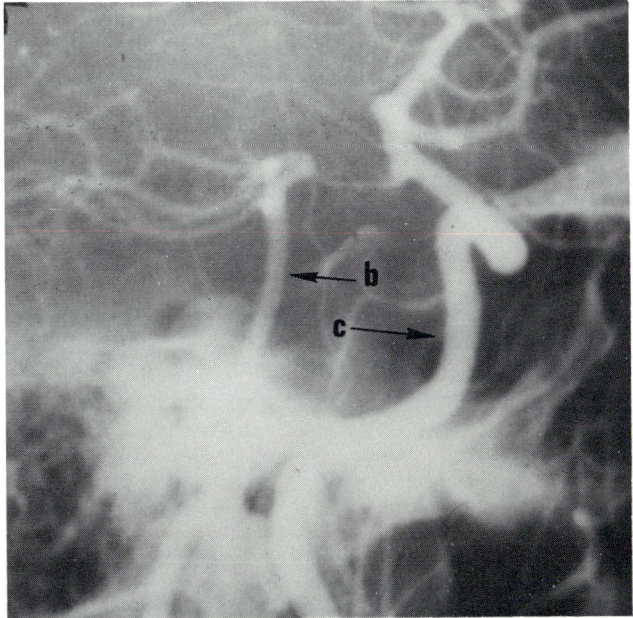

Fig. 5-8. Clivus chordoma. Right brachial angiogram, arterial phase, lateral projection (non-subtracted film). The petrous segment of the internal carotid artery (c) is displaced anteriorly, and the basilar artery (b) is displaced posteriorly.

displaced posterosuperiorly have also been seen in acoustic neurinomas (Figs. 5-12, 5-16A,B).[37,38] Arteriovenous shunts may be seen with acoustic neurinomas (Figs. 5-14, 5-15).[36,39,40] In fifth nerve neurinomas, spotty accumulation of contrast material within the tumor has been described, as have abnormal tumor vessels.[19,41]

Elevation of the superior cerebellar artery and the posterior cerebral artery by a tumor mass in the cerebellopontine angle will occur if there is superiorly directed tumor growth (Figs. 5-4, 5-10, 5-17, 5-19).[15,33,35,38,42,43] The superior cerebellar artery is displaced posteriorly and medially if the mass is located anterior or anterolateral to the upper brainstem.[44-46] The typical displacement is that of a superiorly arched marginal branch of the superior cerebellar artery.[35,44] Fifth cranial nerve neurinomas characteristically produce posterior displacement of the superior cerebellar artery and downward displacement of the anterior inferior cerebellar artery.[44] The tumor also displaces the lateral mesencephalic vein posteriorly and increases the space between it and the anterior ponto-mesencephalic vein.[36] Cerebellopontine

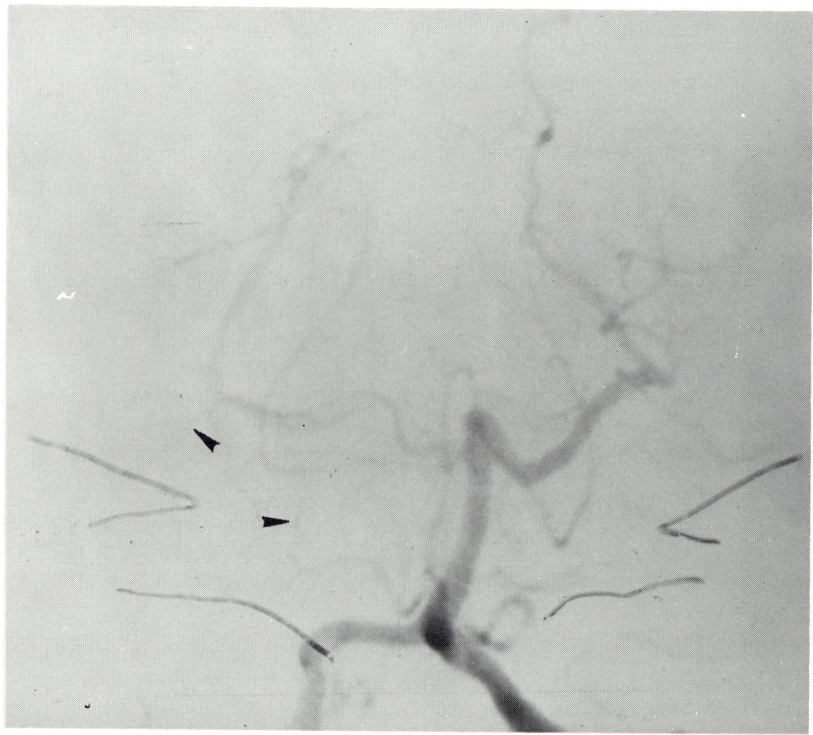

Fig. 5-9. Acoustic neurinoma. Left vertebral angiogram, arterial phase, frontal projection: same case as Figs. 5-10 through 5-12. Note the elevation of the anterior inferior cerebellar artery (arrowheads). (Courtesy A. Robbins, M.D., Veterans Administration Hospital, Boston, Massachusetts.)

angle tumors can cause brainstem rotation that will cause the lateral medullary segment of the posterior inferior cerebellar artery to be displaced toward the normal side. Brainstem rotation will also cause the caudal and cranial loops of the posterior inferior cerebellar artery to be closed or displaced backward (Fig. 5-1A).[35] If the anterolateral surface of the cerebellum is displaced backward by the tumor, an associated rotational force on the cerebellum will cause the vermian branches of the posterior inferior cerebellar artery to be displaced toward the normal side.[33,41]

The basilar artery can be posteriorly and laterally displaced if a cerebellopontine angle tumor extends anterior to the brainstem.[16,35]

Contralateral displacement of the basilar artery is relatively rare in cerebellopontine angle tumors since the tumors cause a brainstem rotation with deviation of the basilar artery to the side of the tumor.[35] The tumors when they

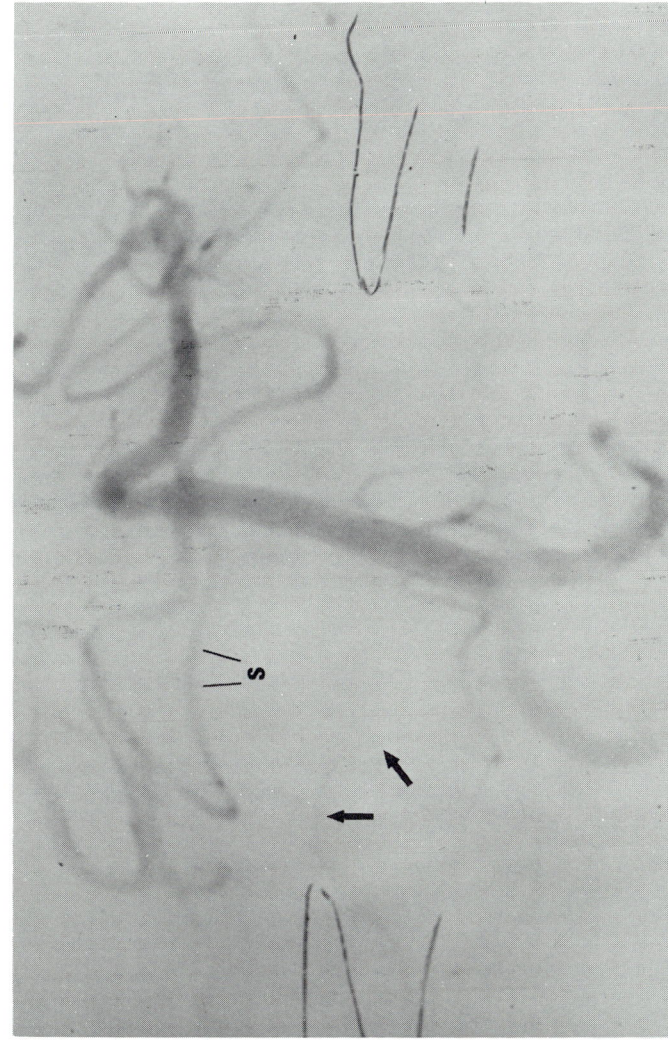

Fig. 5-10. Caldwell projection. The abrupt elevation of the anterior inferior cerebellar artery (arrows) is seen as it is locally displaced by the acoustic neurinoma. The superior cerebellar artery (s) is also elevated. (Courtesy A. Robbins, M.D., Veterans Administration Hospital, Boston, Massachusetts.)

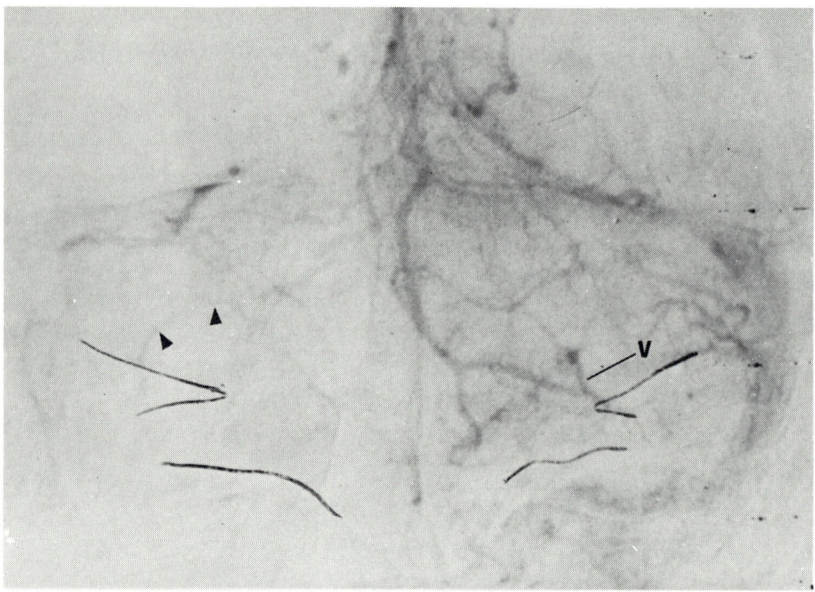

Fig. 5-11. Venous phase, frontal projection. The right petrosal vein (arrowheads) is elevated. The left petrosal vein (v) is in a normal position. (Courtesy A. Robbins, M.D., Veterans Administration Hospital, Boston, Massachusetts.)

are slow growing can burrow into the brainstem and displace the basilar artery anteriorly. We have seen this with meningiomas (Figs. 5-18, 5-19, 5-20) and with acoustic neurinomas.

The diagnostic accuracy of vertebral angiography in acoustic neurinomas appears to be dependent on tumor size. According to Takahashi and associates the diagnostic accuracy is low with tumors below 1.5 cm in diameter, but is considerably higher with tumors greater than 2.0 cm in size.[35]

When a glomus jugulare tumor extends into the cerebellopontine angle, vertebral angiography will demonstrate the presence of a mass lesion indistinguishable from a meningioma or an acoustic neurinoma. The presence of a blood supply derived from the ascending pharyngeal artery, with occlusion of the jugular vein on venography, and the typical irregular erosion of the jugular foramen, however, should allow the correct diagnosis to be made.[47] Meningeal branches of the external carotid artery and the vertebral artery may be enlarged with glomus jugulare tumors.[25,47] Occasionally, glomus jugulare tumors involving the tympanum may derive their blood supply from the meningo-

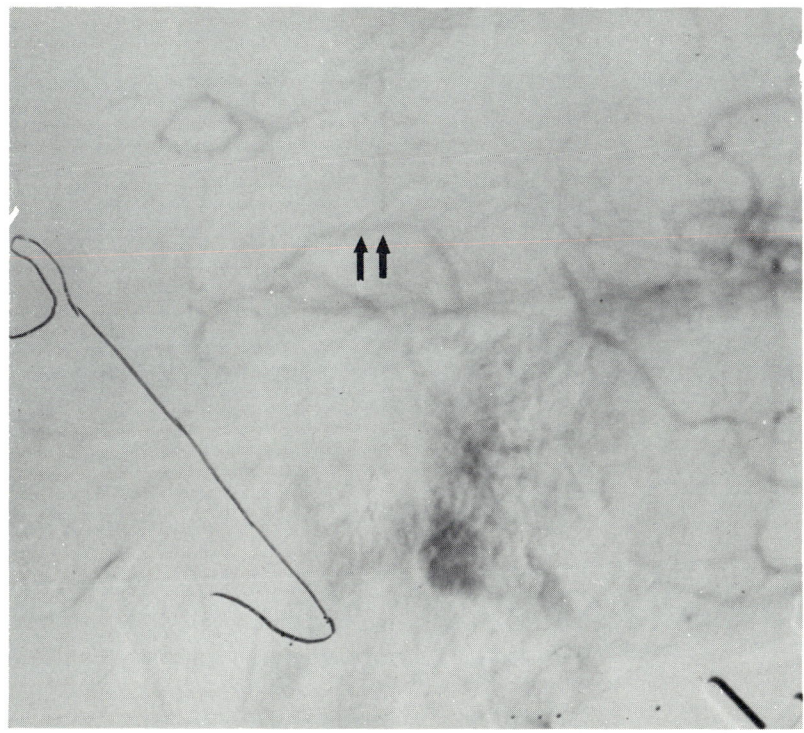

Fig. 5-12. Venous phase, lateral projection. Elevation of veins above the petrous bone is seen (arrows). (Courtesy A. Robbins, M.D., Veterans Administration Hospital, Boston, Massachusetts.)

hyophyseal artery or the caroticotympanic artery.[48]* The investigation of these patients, therefore, must include internal carotid angiography. Infrequently, glomus jugulare tumors may have the angiographic appearance of an irregular network of small vessels with pooling of contrast material in vascular "lakes" with an arteriovenous shunt.[49]

Neurinomas of the cranial nerves nine, ten, or eleven can cause angiographic characteristics indistinguishable from other more common cerebellopontine angle tumors (Fig. 5-17).

The angiographic changes in epidermoids have recently been described. Characteristically, they are avascular tumors and cause changes in the anterior

---

*The caroticotympanic artery originates from the petrous portion of the internal carotid artery to enter the tympanic cavity.[50]

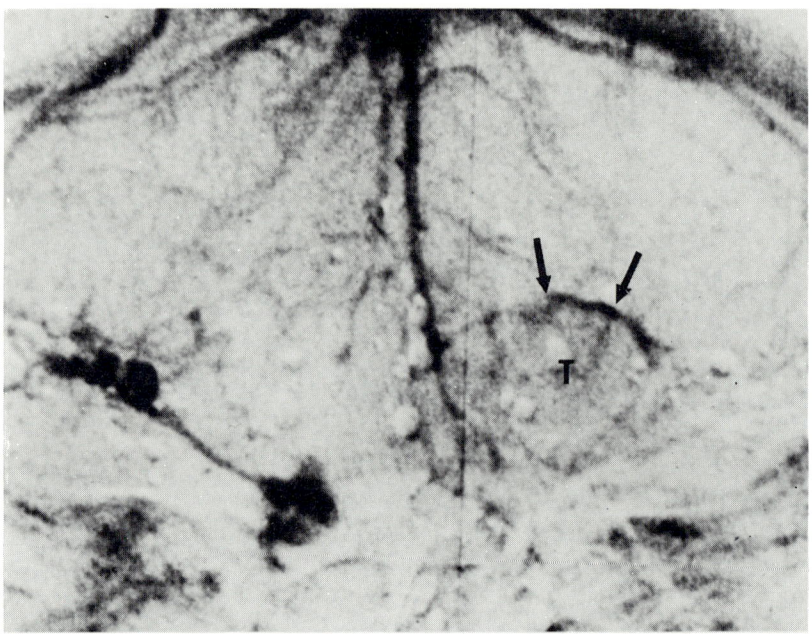

Fig. 5-13. Acoustic neurinoma. Left vertebral angiogram, venous phase, frontal projection. The left petrosal vein is elevated (arrows). A tumor stain (T) is also present. The stain was maximally seen in the venous phase.

inferior cerebellar artery and petrosal vein indistinguishable from the more common cerebellopontine angle tumors.[51]

RETROCEREBELLAR EXTRA-AXIAL TUMORS

Tumors in this group are very rare. Congenital arachnoid cysts are the most common tumors and, characteristically, displace all the arterial and venous branches of the cerebellum anteriorly away from the cerebellum. The torcula and transverse sinuses are elevated since the cysts have developed embryologically prior to the fixation of the venous sinuses to the calvarium.[52] Dermoid cysts and fibromas may also occur in this location.

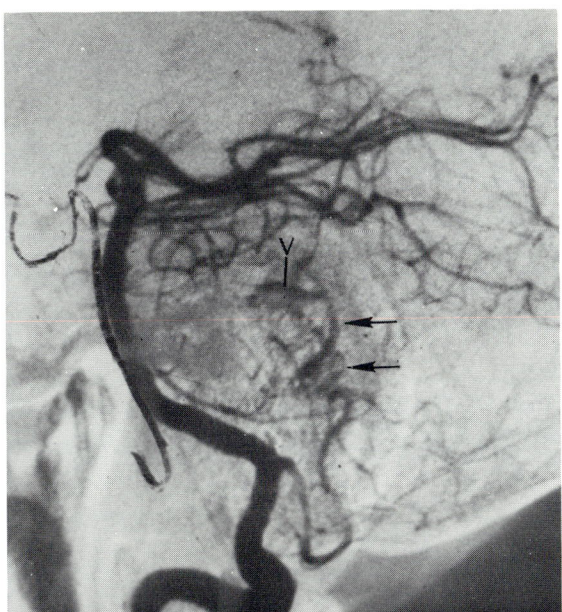

Fig. 5-14. Acoustic neurinoma. Left vertebral angiogram, arterial phase, lateral projection: Same case as Figs. 5-15, 5-16A,B. An arteriovenous shunt is present (arrows). The draining vein (v) is enlarged.

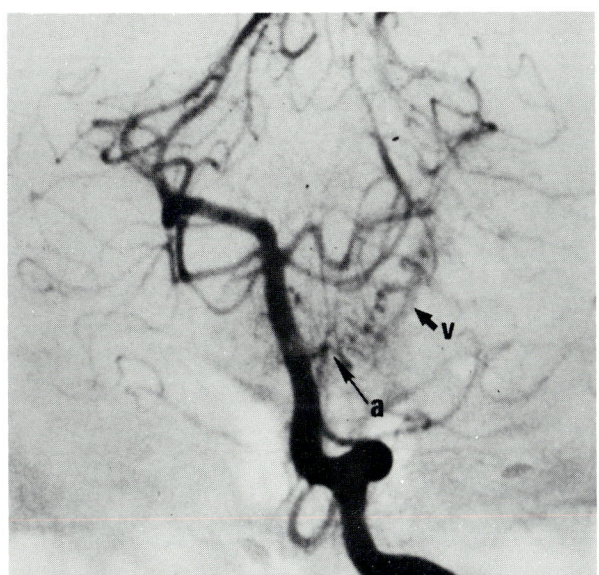

Fig. 5-15. Frontal projection. The anterior inferior cerebellar artery (a) is enlarged. A shunt into an early draining vein (v) is present. A faint tumor stain is also apparent.

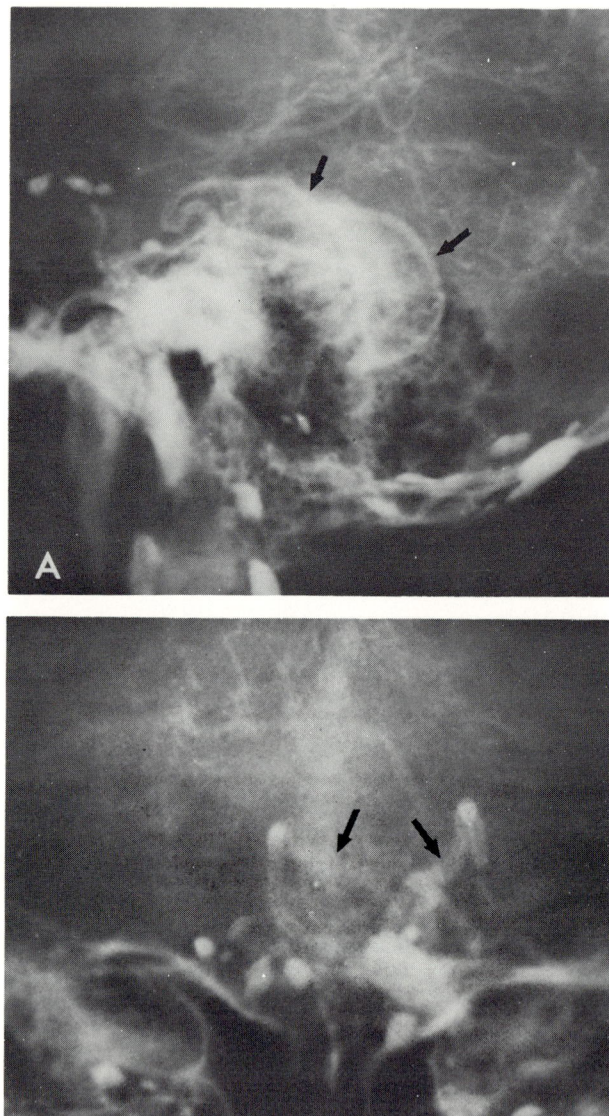

Fig. 5-16A,B. Venous phase, lateral and frontal projections (non-subtracted films). The enlarged draining veins are seen surrounding the tumor (arrows).

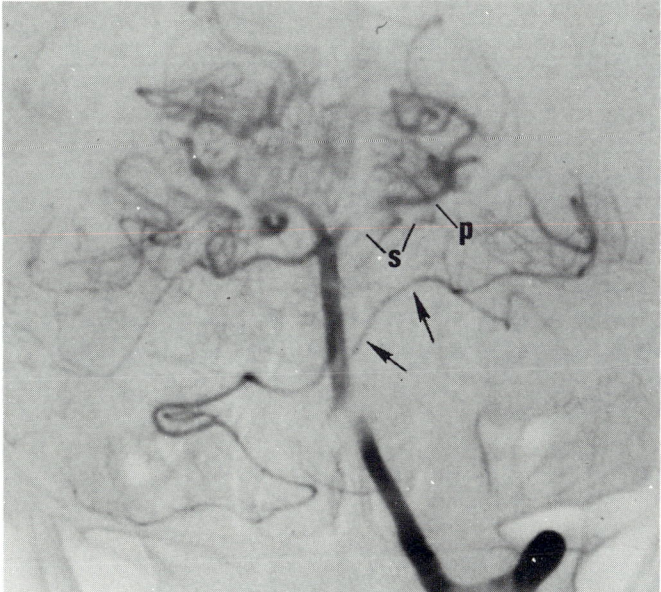

Fig. 5-17. A ninth nerve neurinoma. Left vertebral angiogram, arterial phase, frontal projection. There is elevation of the anterior inferior cerebellar artery (arrows). The superior cerebellar artery (s) and the posterior cerebral artery (p) are also elevated on the side of the lesion.

REFERENCES

1. Pool JL, Pava AA, Greenfield EC: Acoustic Nerve Tumors Early Diagnosis and Treatment (ed 2). Springfield, Charles C Thomas, 1970
2. Bull J: Massive aneurysms at the base of the brain. Brain 92:535, 1969
3. Scatliff JH, Kier EL, Zingesser LH, et al: Terminal basilar artery deformity secondary to suprasellar masses and third ventricular dilatation. Am J Roentgenol 101:61, 1967
4. Plaut HF, Blatt ES: Chordoma of the clivus. A report of four cases. Am J Roentgenol 100:639, 1967
5. Solomon GE, Tolge BP, Palesty J, Waltner JC, Potter GD: An extra-axial brainstem tumor of childhood. Am J Dis Child 117:338, 1969
6. Harwood-Nash DC: The radiology of rhabdomyosarcomas of the middle ear with intracranial extension in children. Clin Radiol 22:321, 1971
7. Hitselberger WE, Gardner G, Jr: Other tumors of the cerebellopontine angle. Arch Otolaryngol 88:712, 1968
8. Hitselberger WE, Hughes RL: Bilateral acoustic tumors and neurofibromatosis. Arch Otolaryngol 88:700, 1968

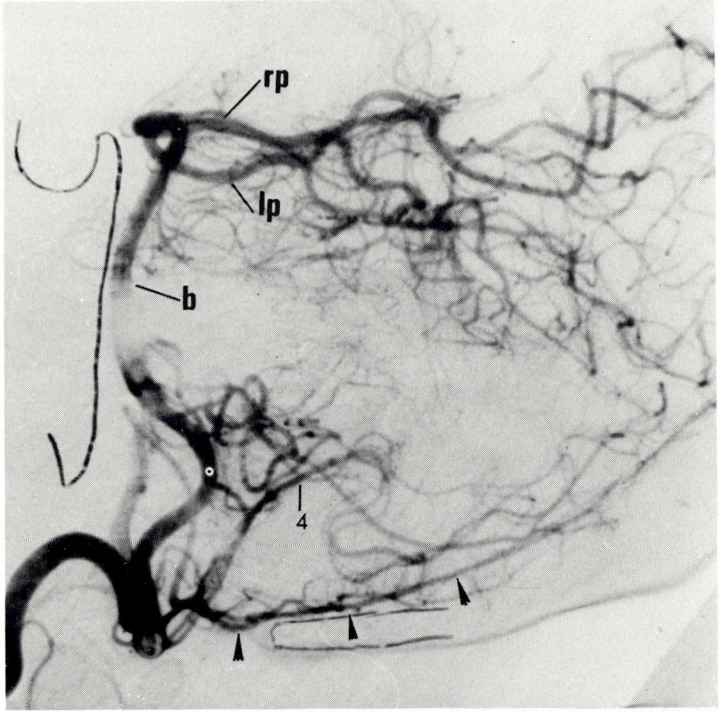

Fig. 5-18. Cerebellopontine angle meningioma. Left vertebral angiogram, arterial phase, lateral projection: Same case as Figs. 5-19, 5-20. The basilar artery (b) is slightly anteriorly displaced toward the clivus. The ambient segment (rp) of the right posterior cerebral artery is elevated compared with the equivalent segment (lp) of the left posterior cerebral artery. The supratonsillar segments (4) of both PICAs are superimposed and displaced posteroinferiorly with effacement of the adjacent choroidal points. Note the posterior meningeal branch of the vertebral artery (arrowheads).

9. Davidoff LM, Martin J: Hereditary combined neurinomas and meningomas. J Neurosurg 12:375, 1955
10. Castellano F, Ruggiero G: Meningiomas of the posterior fossa. Acta Radiol (Suppl) (Stockh) 104, 1953
11. Danziger J, Lewer-Allen K, Bloch S: Intracranial chordomas. Clin Radiol 25:309, 1974
12. Schechter MM, Liebeskind AL, Azar-Kia B: Intracranial chordomas. Neuroradiology 8:67, 1974
13. Falconer MA, Bailey IC, Duchen LW: Surgical treatment of chordoma and chondroma of the skull base. J Neurosurg 29:261, 1968
14. Taveras JM, Wood EH: Diagnostic Neuroradiology. Baltimore, Williams & Wilkins, 1964

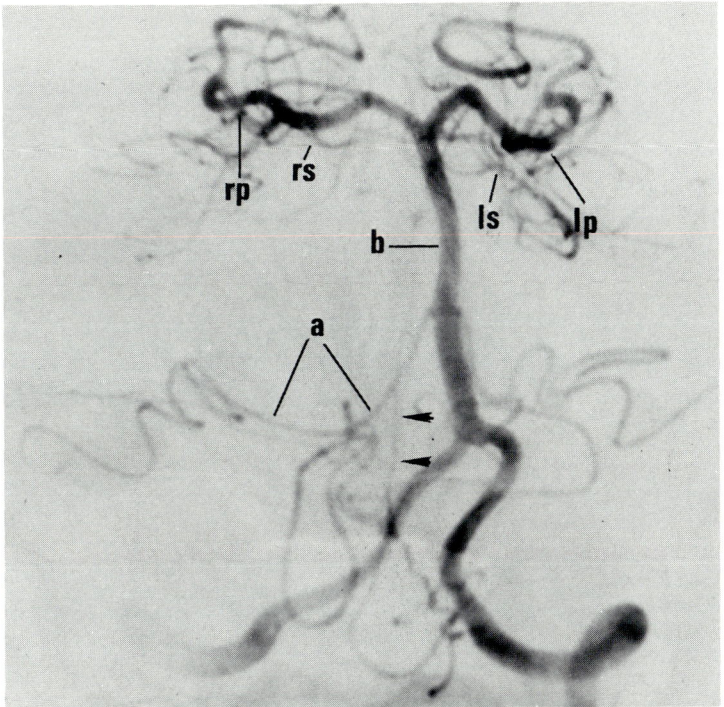

Fig. 5-19. Caldwell projection. The basilar artery (b) is displaced to the left side. The ambient segment (rp) of the right posterior cerebral artery is elevated as compared with the equivalent segment (lp) of the left side. The ambient segment (rs) of the right superior cerebellar artery is similarly elevated as compared with the ambient segment (ls) on the left side. The anterior inferior cerebellar artery (a) is stretched and displaced inferiorly. Both PICAs are unremarkable. The appearances in conjunction with lateral displacement of the petrosal vein (not shown) indicate an extra-axial mass lesion. Note the posterior meningeal branch of the vertebral artery (arrowheads).

15. Dufour M, Legré J: Aspects Neuro-radiologiques du diagnostic des tumeurs de la fosse postérieure. Ann Radiol (Paris) 12:473, 1969
16. Lang ER, Watts JW, Jakoby RK, Fox JL: Recent observations on the diagnosis and pathologic anatomy of posterior fossa meningiomas. Johns Hopkins Med J 122:336, 1968
17. Galligioni F, Bernardi R, Pellone M, Iraci G: The veins of the posterior cranial fossa: an angiographic study under pathologic conditions. Am J Roentgenol 110:39, 1970
18. Salamon GM, Combalbert A, Raybaud C, Gonzalez J: An angiographic study of meningiomas of the posterior fossa. J Neurosurg 35:731, 1971
19. Westberg G: Angiographic changes in neurinoma of the trigeminal nerve. Acta Radiol [Diagn] (Stockh) 1:513, 1963

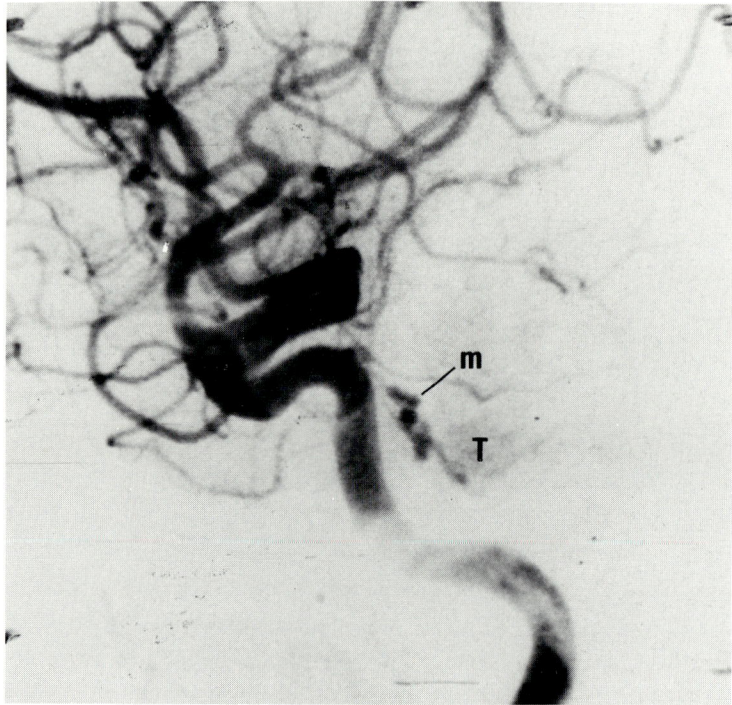

Fig. 5-20. Left carotid angiogram arterial phase, lateral projection. The meningohypophyseal trunk (m) is enlarged and ends in a tumor stain (T).

The appearances of the vertebral angiogram could indicate an intrinsic pontine glioma with an exophytic component growing into the cerebellopontine angle cistern. The primary blood supply from the dural branches, however, suggests the extra-axial origin of the tumor.

20. Wallace S, Goldberg HI, Leeds NE, Mishkin MM: The cavernous branches of the internal carotid artery. Am J Roentgenol 101:34, 1967
21. Théron J, Lasjaunias P: Participation of the external and internal carotid arteries in the vascular supply of cerebellopontine angle tumours. Thirteenth Annual Meeting of American Society of Neuroradiology, Vancouver, B.C., 1975
22. Radner S: Vertebral angiography by catheterization. A new method employed in 221 cases. Acta Radiol (Suppl) (Stockh) 87, 1951
23. Minagi H, Newton TH: Cartilaginous tumors of the base of skull. Am J Roentgenol 105:308, 1969
24. Newton TH: The anterior and posterior meningeal branches of the vertebral artery. Radiology 91:271, 1968

25. Greitz T, Laurén T: Anterior meningeal branch of the vertebral artery. Acta Radiol [Diagn] (Stockh) 7:219, 1968
26. Morris MB: Anterior meningeal branch of vertebral artery. Br J Radiol 42:308, 1969
27. Pachtman H, Waldron R, II: Anterior meningeal branch of the vertebral artery in extra-axial posterior fossa lesions. Am J Roentgenol 122:545, 1974
28. Kendall B, Shah S: Investigation of meningiomas of cerebellar convexities. Neuroradiology 4:162, 1972
29. Takahashi M, Wilson G, Hanafee W: The anterior inferior cerebellar artery: its radiographic anatomy and significance in the diagnosis of extra-axial tumors of the posterior fossa. Radiology 90:281, 1968
30. Handa H, Handa J, Koyama T: Agenesis of the Corpus Callosum associated with multiple developmental anomalies of the cerebral arteries: report of a case and review of the literature. Brain Nerve (Tokyo) 20:317, 1968
31. Takahashi M: The anterior inferior cerebellar artery, in Newton TH, Potts DG (eds): Radiology of the Skull and Brain, vol 2, book 2. St. Louis, Mosby, 1974, p 1796
32. Smaltino F, Bernini FP, Elefante R: Normal and pathological findings of the angiographic examination of the internal auditory artery. Neuroradiology 2:216, 1971
33. Takahashi M, Wilson G, Hanafee W: The significance of the petrosal vein in the diagnosis of cerebellopontine angle tumors. Radiology 89:834, 1967
34. Bull J, Kozlowski P: The angiographic pattern of the petrosal veins in the normal and pathological. Neuroradiology 1:20, 1970
35. Takahashi M, Okudera T, Tomanaga M, Kitamura K: Angiographic diagnosis of acoustic neurinomas: analysis of 30 lesions. Neuroradiology 2:191, 1971
36. Symon L, Kendall B: The use of vertebral angiography in the differential diagnosis of cerebello-pontine angle lesions, in Schürmann K, Brock M, Reulen H, Voth D (eds): Advances in Neurosurgery, vol 1. Berlin, Springer-Verlag, 1973
37. Mani RL, Newton TH, Glickman MG: The superior cerebellar artery: an anatomic roentgenographic correlation. Radiology 91:1102, 1968
38. Des Plantes ZBG: X-Ray examination in cerebellopontine angle tumours. Psychiatr Neurol Neurochir 71:133, 1968
39. King CD, Long JM, Hammon WB: Early draining veins in acoustic neurinomas. Radiology 113:369, 1974
40. Moscow NP, Newton TH: Angiographic features of hypervascular neurinomas of the head and neck. Radiology 114:635, 1975
41. Hauge T: Catheter vertebral Angiography. Acta Radiol (Suppl) (Stockh) 109, 1954
42. Goree JA, Tindall GE, Odom GL: Percutaneous retrograde brachial angiography in the diagnosis of acoustic neurinoma. Results in 4 cases. Am J Roentgenol 92:829, 1964
43. Olsson O: Vertebral angiography in diagnosis of acoustic nerve tumours. Acta Radiol 139:265, 1953
44. Mani RL, Newton TH: The superior cerebellar artery: arteriographic changes in the diagnosis of posterior fossa lesions. Radiology 92:1281, 1969
45. Khilnani M, Silverstein A: Displacement of the superior cerebellar artery. A means of distinguishing intra- and extra-axial posterior fossa masses by vertebral arteriography. Arch Neurol 8:502, 1963
46. Economos D, Prosalentis A: L'artère Cerebelleuse superieure dans les tumeurs de la Fosse Posterieure. Acta Radiol [Diagn] (Stockh) 1:267, 1963
47. Palacios E: Chemodectomas of the head and neck. Am J Roentgenol 110:129, 1970
48. Jordan CE, Newton TH: Internal carotid artery supply to temporal bone chemodectomas. Neuroradiology 8:253, 1975

49. Hawkins TD: Glomus jugulare and carotid body tumours. Clin Radiol 12:199, 1961
50. Gray H: Gray's Anatomy (ed 28) Philadelphia, Lea & Febiger, 1966
51. Long JM, Kier EL, Schechter MM: The radiology of epidermoid tumors of the cerebellopontine angle. Neuroradiology 6:188, 1973
52. Wolpert SM, Haller JS, Rabe EF: The value of angiography in the Dandy-Walker syndrome and posterior fossa extra-axial cysts. Am J Roentgenol 109:261, 1970

6
Pontine and Mesencephalic Tumors (Plate IV*)

The most common brainstem tumor is a low-grade glial tumor such as an astrocytoma.[1] Less frequently, glioblastomas multiforme, oliogodendrogliomas or metastases may occur in the brainstem. Characteristically, the gliomas are slow-growing and present clinically with cranial nerve and long tract signs before signs of hydrocephalus occur. The tumors can originate in the pons, the medulla, or the midbrain and, frequently, the exact site of origin cannot be determined.

Expansion of the pons can occur anteriorly, laterally, or posteriorly. In evaluating the angiographic signs of pontine expansion, it is convenient to consider the arterial and venous displacements in light of the different directions of expansion. In any one case, however, expansion frequently occurs in all three directions as well as superiorly and inferiorly, and the angiographic findings may then include some or all of the following changes (Table 6-1).

Anterior Displacements

These displacements are appreciated in the lateral projection. The basilar artery and pontine segment of the ponto-mesencephalic vein are characteristically displaced anteriorly.[1-3] These changes, however, are nonspecific and occur with any intrinsic mass lesion posterior to these vessels. It is possible, however, for the basilar artery and ponto-mesencephalic vein to be posteriorly displaced and the transverse pontine veins anteriorly displaced (Figs. 6-1,

*See color plate, page 34.

Table 6-1
Differential Diagnosis of Pontine from Fourth Ventricle Tumors

	Displacements	
Anatomical Location	Pontine Tumors	Fourth Ventricle Tumors
Arteries		
Basilar	Anterior Posterior (exophytic)	Anterior
Posterior inferior cerebellar		
Lateral medullary	Stretched—minimal lateral	Lateral if medulla is compressed
Posterior medullary	Posterior	Minimal anterior, may be posterior
Supratonsillar	Posterior—not lateral	Lateral with stretching
Retrotonsillar	Posterior—not lateral	Lateral and posterior
Choroidal point	Posterior	Variable
Superior cerebellar		
Ambient	Stretched with midbrain involvement	Uninvolved
Superior vermian	Uninvolved	Superior and posterior if tumor has extended into superior vermis
Veins		
Pontine	Anterior Posterior (exophytic)	Anterior
Lateral recess	Minimal lateral or medial	Anterior and marked lateral
Precentral cerebellar	Posterior with increase in colliculo-central angle	Posterior with decrease in colliculo-central angle Anterior if tumor has extended into superior vermis

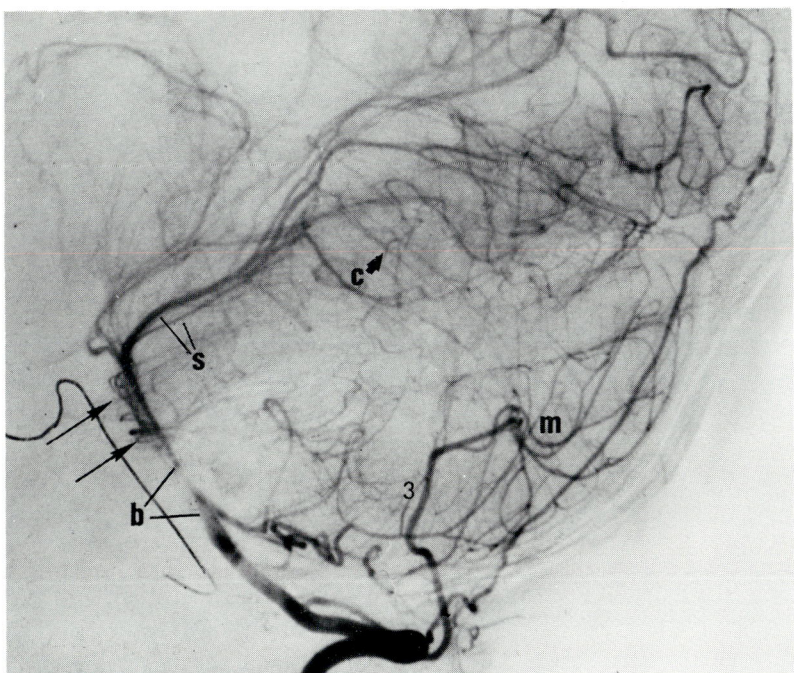

Fig. 6-1. Pontine glioma. Left vertebral angiogram, arterial phase, lateral projection: same cases as Figs. 6-2 through 6-5. The basilar artery (b) is slightly separated from the clivus, and hypertrophied pontine arteries (arrows) are seen to extend anterior to the basilar artery. This indicates envelopment of the basilar artery by the tumor. There is some posterior displacement of the upper part of the posterior medullary segment (3) of the posterior inferior cerebellar artery. The copular point (m) is also displaced posteriorly. The crural segment of the superior cerebellar artery (s) has lost its normal convex inferior curve. The precentral cerebellar artery (c) (identified by comparing with the precentral cerebellar vein in Fig. 6-2) is posteriorly displaced.

6-2).[1] This paradoxical combination of appearances is due to nodular hypertrophy of the surface of the enlarged pons with consequent envelopment of the basilar artery and ponto-mesencephalic vein.[4,5] The basilar artery is then displaced away from the clivus, but more laterally located pontine veins lying ventral to the nodular hypertrophy are displaced anteriorly.[1] Alternatively, if the nodular hypertrophy envelops the ponto-mesencephalic vein, the vein can be posteriorly displaced, whereas the basilar artery that does not adhere to the anterior aspect of the pons can be anteriorly displaced.[6]

The transverse pontine arteries can be hypertrophied and stretched. If the basilar artery is enveloped by the tumor, the pontine arteries are projected anterior to the basilar artery (Fig. 6-1).

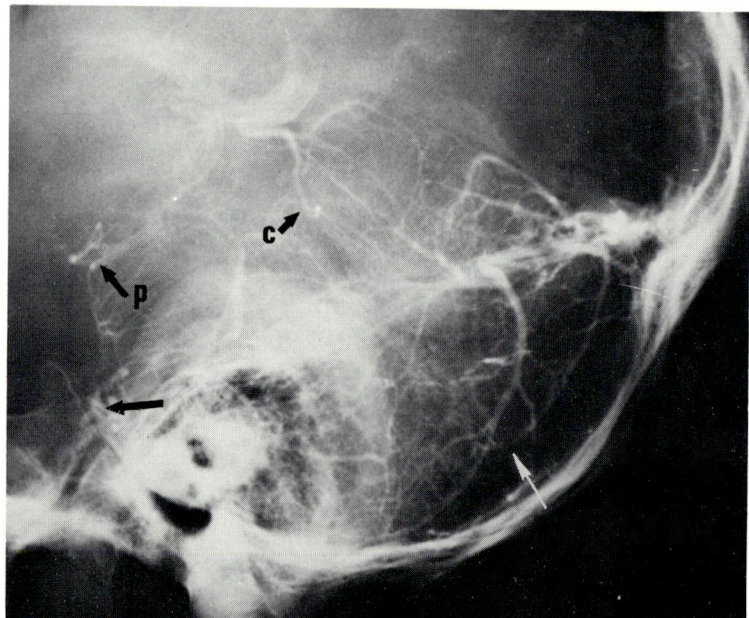

Fig. 6-2. Venous phase, lateral projection (non-subtracted film). The pontine segment (arrow) of the ponto-mesencephalic vein is anteriorly displaced, and the mesencephalic segment (p) is elevated. The precentral cerebellar vein (c) is posteriorly displaced. The copular point (white arrow) is posteriorly displaced.

When the midbrain is involved, the mesencephalic segment of the ponto-mesencephalic vein is elevated due to compression of the interpeduncular cistern from below (Fig. 6-2).[1]

With medullary involvement, the anterior spinal artery is anteriorly displaced.[7]

Lateral Displacements

These displacements are best appreciated in the semiaxial projection. When the tumor involves the lower brainstem, the lateral medullary segment of the posterior inferior cerebellar artery may be stretched and laterally displaced.[8] Due to the potential for variations in this segment, however, where it can normally extend laterally and inferiorly into the medullary cistern, lateral displacement may not be present.[1] It would be expected that the vein of the lateral recess of the fourth ventricle, which lies lateral to the medulla, would always be laterally displaced in lower brainstem and medullary tumors (Fig. 6-4). Since the tumor, however, not infrequently involves the brachium pontis

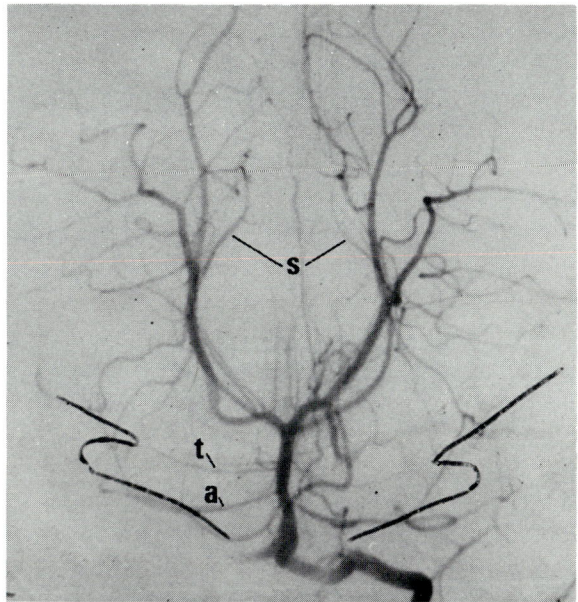

Fig. 6-3. Arterial phase, frontal projection. The anterior inferior cerebellar artery (a) and a transverse pontine artery (t) on the right side are stretched. The ambient and quadrigeminal segments of the superior cerebellar artery (s) are separated.

and restiform body, which normally lie lateral to the vein, the vein might not be displaced (Fig. 6-13).[1]

Hypertrophy and stretching of the transverse pontine arteries and stretching of the anterior inferior cerebellar arteries indicate lateral expansion of the pons in the frontal projection (Figs. 6-3, 6-5).

When the tumor involves the midbrain, the ambient segment of the superior cerebellar artery is laterally displaced, increasing the curvature of this vessel in the semiaxial projection (Fig. 6-3).[9] Furthermore, the normal downward dipping of the artery as seen on the lateral projection is lost, and the artery extends directly posteriorly from the basilar artery (Fig. 6-1).[1] The lateral anastomotic mesencephalic vein, when present, is laterally displaced (Fig. 6-4). Together with the lateral displacement and elevation of the superior cerebellar artery, there may be similar changes in the ambient segment of the posterior cerebral artery (Fig. 6-3).

Lateral displacement of the ambient segments of the superior cerebellar and posterior cerebral arteries is not invariably seen. If there is exophytic extension of a midbrain glioma into the ambient cistern, there may be paradoxi-

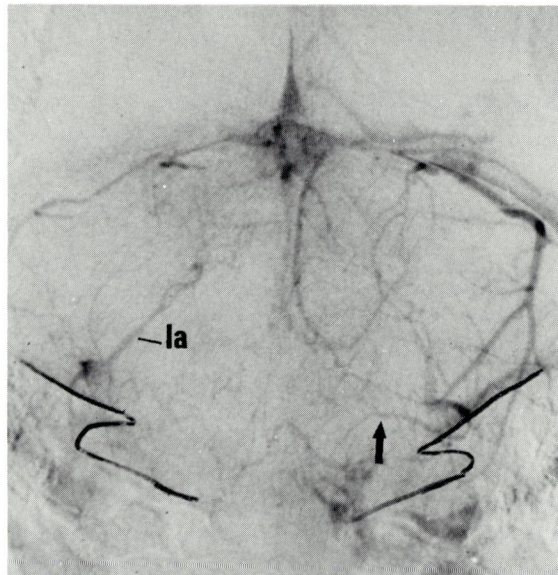

Fig. 6-4. Venous phase, frontal projection. The vein of the lateral recess of the fourth ventricle (arrow) is tilted backward due to tumor extending into the cerebellomedullary fissure. The lateral anastomotic mesencephalic vein (1a) is laterally displaced, indicating involvement of the brachium pontis.

cal medial displacement of the superior cerebellar artery and the posterior mesencephalic vein.[1]

With exophytic extension of a pontine glioma into the cerebellopontine angle cistern, the differential diagnosis from a primary fourth ventricle tumor with similar exophytic growth may be extremely difficult due to the combination of angiographic changes seen in both cases. The diagnosis may then depend entirely on the position of the vein of the lateral recess of the fourth ventricle. As already described (p. 118), if the vein is not laterally displaced, this favors a pontine tumor, whereas lateral displacement of the vein favors a fourth ventricle tumor (see also p. 134).

The posterior mesencephalic vein and the basal vein of Rosenthal may be displaced superiorly and laterally with high midbrain tumors.

Posterior Displacements

Posterior displacements can be appreciated in the lateral projection. With a low brainstem tumor, the posterior medullary segment of the posterior inferior cerebellar artery lying behind and lateral to the medulla is displaced

Pontine and Mesencephalic Tumors

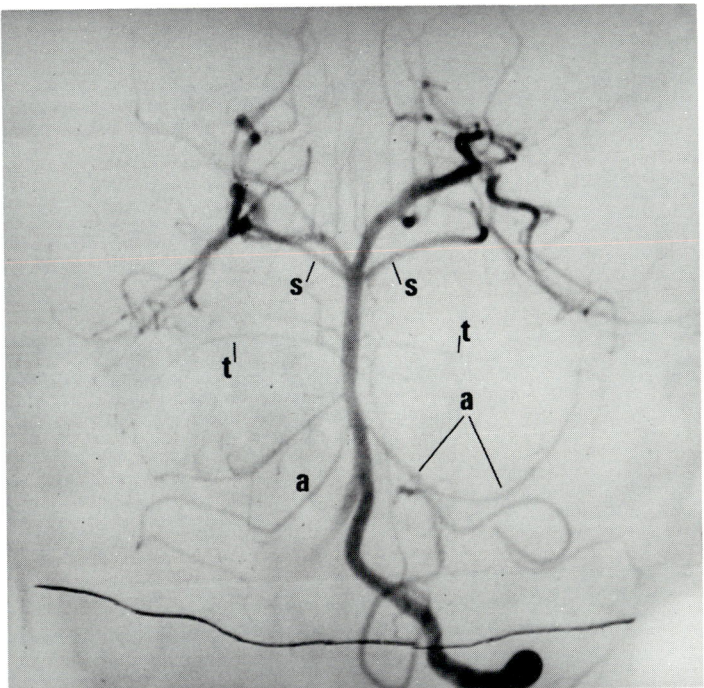

Fig. 6-5. Arterial phase, Caldwell projection. The anterior inferior cerebellar arteries (a) and the transverse pontine arteries (t) are stretched. The crural segments of the superior cerebellar arteries (s) are also stretched.

posteriorly (Figs. 6.1, 6-6, 6-7). The choroid arch is also posteriorly displaced.[1,10,11] Depending on whether the tonsil is involved by the tumor or not, the distance between the posterior medullary segment and the retrotonsillar segment of PICA is maintained or diminished. Similarly, the copula pyramidal loop of the inferior vermian branch of the posterior inferior cerebellar artery will be widened or compressed, depending on whether or not tumor is present in the tonsil.

A low brainstem tumor will displace the copular point of the inferior vermian vein posteriorly (Fig. 6-2).[1] If the tributaries of the vein of the lateral recess of the fourth ventricle lying above and below the tonsil are identified, they are seen to be displaced posteriorly.

In a high brainstem tumor, there is posterior displacement of both the precentral cerebellar artery and vein (Figs. 6-1, 6-2).[1] The artery, which is a branch of the superior cerebellar artery, is more difficult to identify than the vein, but angiotomography is helpful. With the posterior displacement of the precentral cerebellar vein, there is an increase in the colliculo-central angle.

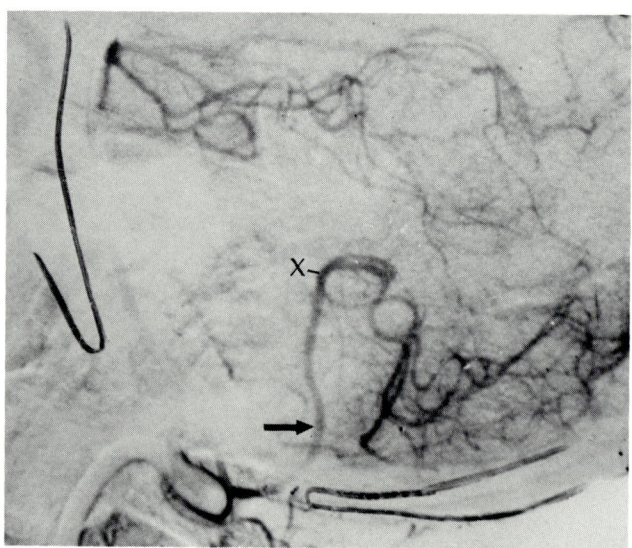

Fig. 6-6. Pontine glioma with major involvement of the medulla. Left vertebral angiogram, arterial phase, lateral projection: same case as Fig. 6-7. The posterior medullary segment (arrow) of the posterior inferior cerebellar artery is posteriorly displaced. Compare with Fig. 6-7. The choroidal point (X) is also posteriorly displaced.

Savoiardo and Vaghi reported on the angiographic changes found in a series of 17 brainstem tumors.[12] They found that an increase in the distance between the precentral cerebellar vein (colliculo-central point) and the anterior ponto-mesencephalic vein (Normal 18 to 23 mm; see p. 82) was the most reliable sign of an upper brainstem tumor. With lower brainstem tumors, posterior displacement of the choroidal point measured off Twining's line (Normal 53 to 59 percent; see p. 46) was the most reliable sign.

Often, brainstem gliomas are eccentric, involving one-half of the brainstem.[5] Under these circumstances, comparison of the angiographic appearances between the two sides of the brainstem is of major importance.[13] With eccentric low brainstem tumors, the posterior medullary segment of the posterior inferior cerebellar artery shows greater posterior displacement on the abnormal side. Depending on the tumor size, similar eccentric displacement involves the copular points of the inferior vermian artery and inferior vermian vein.

With eccentric gliomas involving the high brainstem, the transverse pon-

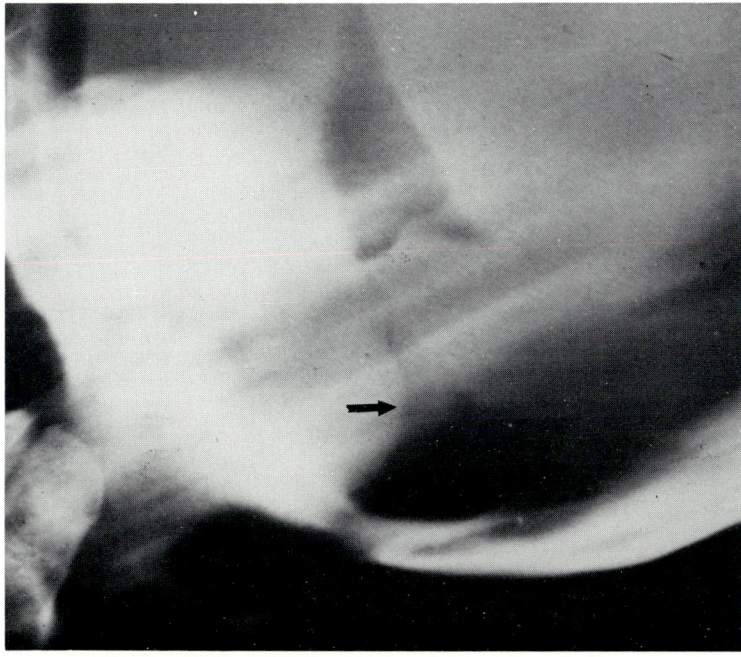

Fig. 6-7. Pneumoencephalography demonstrates involvement of the medulla by the tumor (arrow).

tine veins will be displaced anteriorly on the side of the lesion. This can best be appreciated on the semiaxial projection. The perimesencephalic portion of the superior cerebellar artery and the posterior mesencephalic veins are also displaced further laterally on the side of greater involvement.[9,13]

Rarely, pontine tumors may be highly vascular. We have seen a female, 44 years old, in whom angiography demonstrated a vascular tumor stain in the midbrain. Pathological confirmation, however, was not available.

Angiographically, an acute pontine hemorrhage can mimic a pontine tumor.[14]

QUADRIGEMINAL PLATE TUMORS

Tumors of the quadrigeminal plate consist mainly of gliomas, though pineal tumors can extend inferiorly to infiltrate the quadrigeminal plate. The effect of tumors of the quadrigeminal plate is to compress the anterosuperior

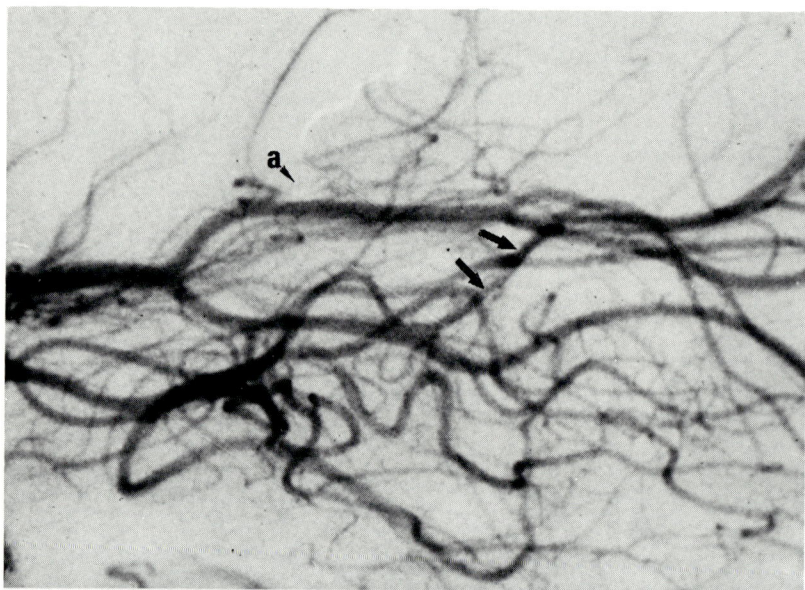

Fig. 6-8. Quadrigeminal plate glioma. Left vertebral angiogram, arterial phase, lateral projection: same case as Figs. 6-9 through 6-12. The quadrigeminal segment (arrows) of the superior cerebellar artery is posteriorly displaced. Previous Pantopaque® ventriculography demonstrated a complete block at the junction of the aqueduct and posterior third ventricle (a).

surface of the vermis, giving it a pointed, instead of a rounded, appearance.[15] As a result, the major angiographic deformity involves the precentral cerebellar vein and the quadrigeminal segment of the superior cerebellar artery. The vein is posteriorly displaced and is usually associated with a localized arcuate deformity (Figs. 6-9, 6-10).[1,15] The colliculo-central angle is reversed with a posterior convex curve. The quadrigeminal segment of the superior cerebellar artery is also posteriorly displaced (Fig. 6-8). Lateral growth of the tumor causes lateral displacement of both the quadrigeminal segment of the superior cerebellar artery and the posterior mesencephalic vein (Figs. 6-11, 6-12). With growth of the tumor superiorly to involve the pineal gland, there is generally posterior-superior displacement of the choroidal vessels.[15,16]

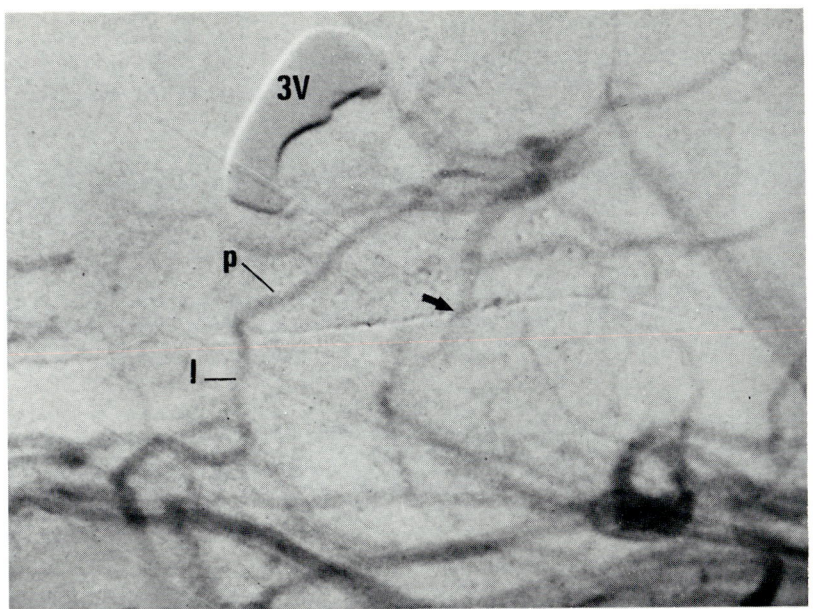

Fig. 6-9. Venous phase, lateral projection. Note the reversal of the normal curve of the precentral cerebellar vein (arrow) and its separation from the third ventricle (3V). The posterior mesesencephalic vein (p) drains into a lateral anastomotic mesencephalic vein (1).

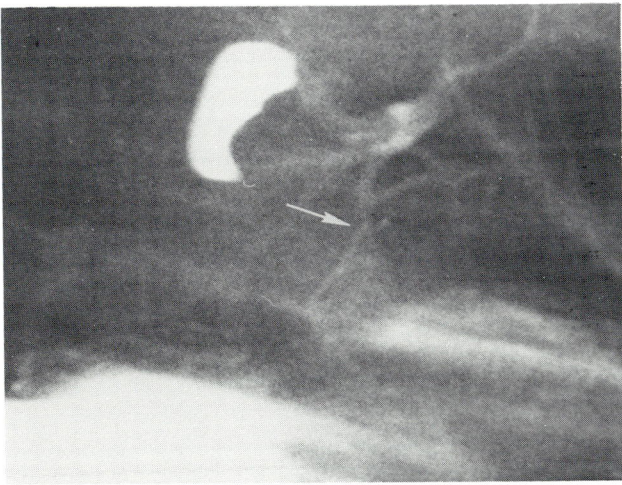

Fig. 6-10. Venous phase, angiotomogram (non-subtracted film). As in Fig. 6-9, the precentral cerebellar vein (white arrow) is posteriorly displaced.

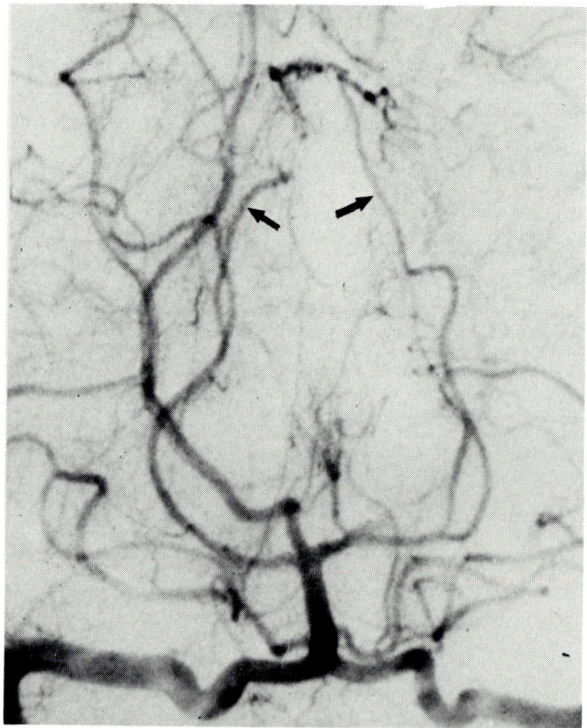

Fig. 6-11. Arterial phase, frontal projection. The quadrigeminal segments (arrows) of the superior cerebellar artery are separated.

REFERENCES

1. Huang YP, Wolf BS: Angiographic features of brain stem tumors and differential diagnosis from fourth ventricle tumors. Am J Roentgenol 110:1, 1970
2. Galligioni F, Bernardi R, Pellone M, Iraci G: The veins of the posterior cranial fossa: an angiographic study under pathologic conditions. Am J Roentgenol 110:39, 1970
3. Dufour M, Legré J: Aspects Neuro-radiologiques du diagnostic des tumeurs de la fosse postérieure. Ann Radiol (Paris) 12:473, 1969
4. Glickman MG, Sholkoff SD: Posterior displacement of the basilar artery by intrinsic pontine tumors. Am J Roentgenol 112:276, 1971
5. Russel DS, Rubinstein LJ: Pathology of Tumours of the Nervous System (ed. 2). London, Arnold, 1963

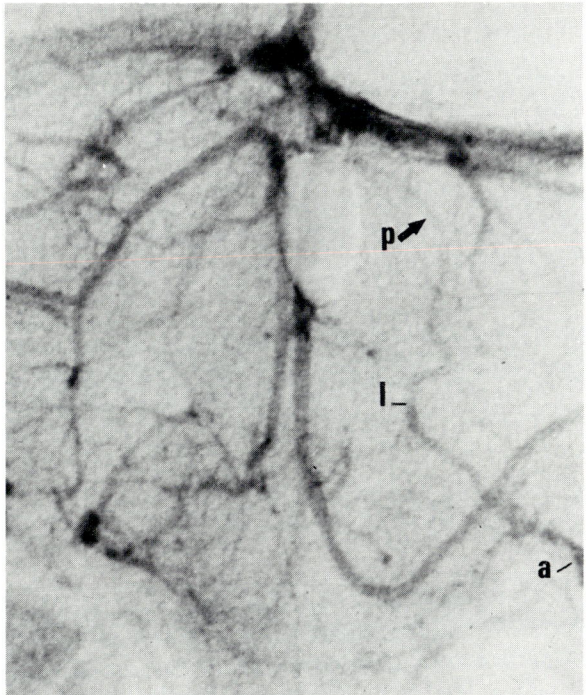

Fig. 6-12. Venous phase, frontal projection. The left posterior mesencephalic vein (p) is laterally displaced. Note its drainage into the lateral anastomotic mesencephalic vein (1) and subsequently the petrosal vein (a).

6. Wackenheim A, BenAmor M: Arteriovenous separation of the prepontine vessels as a sign of intrapontine tumour. Neuroradiology 3:77, 1971
7. Schechter MM, Zingesser L: The spinal arteries. Acta Radiol [Diagn] (Stockh) 5:1124, 1966
8. Takahashi M, Wilson G, Hanafee W: Catheter vertebral angiography: a review of 300 examinations. J Neurosurg 30:722, 1969
9. Economos D, Prosalentis A: L'artère Cerebelleuse superieure dans les tumeurs de la Fosse Posterieure. Acta Radiol [Diagn] (Stockh) 1:267, 1963
10. Peeters FL: Angiography of the vertebral artery in the diagnosis of tumours of the pons cerebelli. A preliminary report. Radiol Clin (Basel) 37:89, 1968
11. Peeters FL: The vertebral angiogram in patients with tumours in or near the midline. Neuroradiology 5:53, 1973
12. Savoiardo M, Vaghi MA: Angiography in brain stem tumors. Neuroradiology 8:99, 1974
13. Seeger JF, Gabrielsen TO: Angiography of eccentric brain stem tumors. Radiology 105:343, 1972

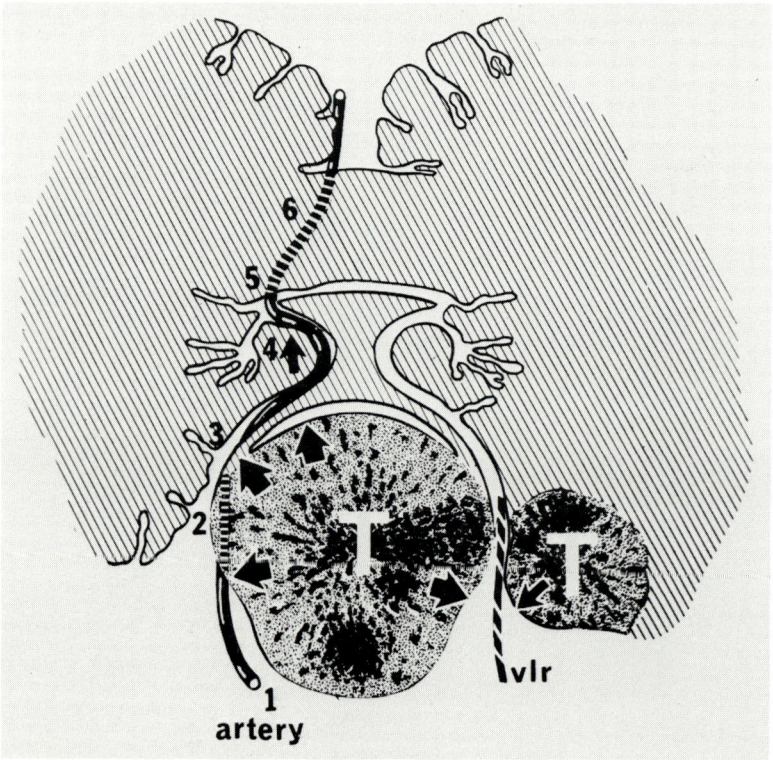

Fig. 6-13. Line diagram of a low pontine tumor. The major arterial displacements are posterior displacement of the posterior medullary (3) and supratonsillar (4) segments of the posterior inferior cerebellar artery. While some lateral displacement of the lateral medullary segment (2) may occur, this is usually minimal as the tumor often involves the adjacent restiform body. Similarly, the vein of the lateral recess (vlr) of the fourth ventricle is often undisplaced. (Compare with Fig. 7-13.)

14. Moscow NP, Margolis MT: Angiography of pontine hemorrhage. Neuroradiology 7:125, 1974
15. Greitz T: Tumours of the quadrigeminal plate and adjacent structures. Acta Radiol [Diagn] (Stockh) 12:513, 1972
16. Wackenheim A, Braun J-P: Angiography of the Mesencephalon; Normal and Pathological Findings. New York, Springer-Verlag, 1970

7
Fourth Ventricle Tumors
(Plate V*)

Fourth ventricle tumors may commence primarily within the fourth ventricle or may be secondary to tumor invasion from adjacent structures. In children and adolescents below the age of 16, 55 percent of all ventricular tumors primarily or secondarily involve the fourth ventricle. In adults, only 20 percent of all intracranial neoplasms involve the fourth ventricle.[1]

According to Koos and Miller, the most common tumor found to involve the fourth ventricle in children is the medulloblastoma.[1] Ependymomas and cerebellar astrocytomas can also present as fourth ventricle tumors. While the ependymomas are almost always primary tumors of the fourth ventricle, the majority of the cerebellar astrocytomas invade the fourth ventricle from the adjacent brain. Rarely, choroid plexus papillomas occur in the fourth ventricle. In adults, involvement of the fourth ventricle most commonly is from displacement by adjacent metastatic or primary tumors of the cerebellum.

Expansion of the fourth ventricle can occur anteriorly, superiorly, inferiorly, and laterally. Angiographic changes can conveniently be considered in the light of vector forces of expansion (see Table 6-1, p. 116). Depending on the size of the tumor, all or some of the following angiographic changes can occur.[2,3]

Anterior Displacements

These are seen on a lateral projection. The basilar artery is displaced anteriorly (Figs. 7-1A, 7-4A, 7-6A). If the tumor is sufficiently large, the

*See color plate, page 34.

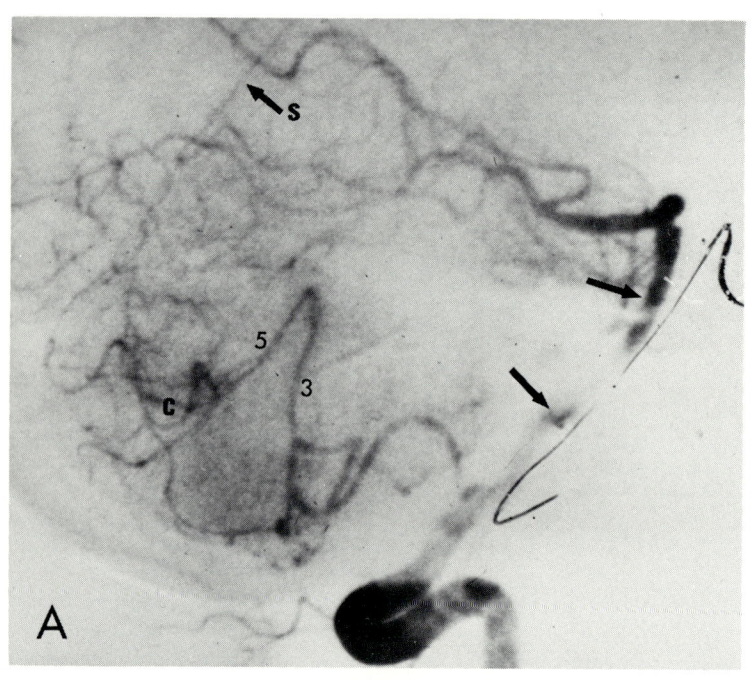
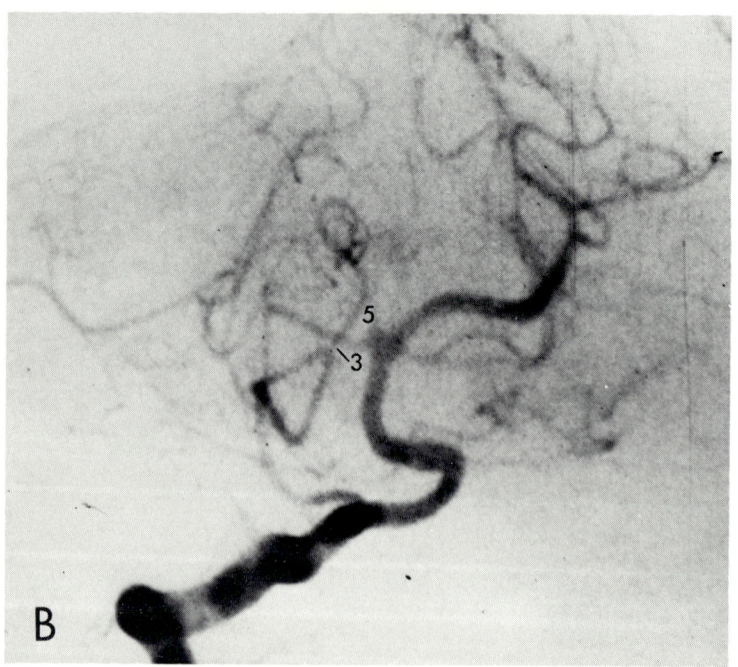

Fourth Ventricle Tumors

pontine segment of the ponto-mesencephalic vein will also be displaced anteriorly (Figs. 7-2, 7-5A). The brainstem is compressed by the enlarged fourth ventricle. As the posterior medullary segment of the posterior inferior cerebellar artery usually lies lateral to, but only slightly anterior to, the fourth ventricle, its anterior displacement is minimal. If the tributaries of the vein of the lateral recess of the fourth ventricle lying above and below the tonsil can be identified on the lateral film, they are seen to be anteriorly displaced.

Superior Displacements

These are seen on a lateral projection. The major superior displacement involves the precentral cerebellar artery and vein. The artery may not be identifiable, but the vein is displaced posteriorly (Fig. 7-2). The vein may also be displaced superiorly, in which case, the angle will be decreased (Fig. 7-11).[4] The superior vermian branches of the superior cerebellar artery and the superior vermian vein (both outlining the superior vermis) are superiorly and posteriorly displaced (Figs. 7-1A, 7-2, 7-4A).

Posterior Displacements

These are seen on a lateral projection. With expansion of the fourth ventricle posteriorly, there is often stretching of the supratonsillar segment of the PICA (Fig. 7-4A). The retrotonsillar segment of the posterior inferior cerebellar artery is posteriorly displaced (Figs. 7-1A, 7-4A). The copular points of the PICA and inferior vermian vein are posteriorly displaced.[5]

On occasions, the posterior medullary segment of the posterior inferior cerebellar artery is posteriorly displaced (Figs. 7-1A, 7-3A, 7-4A). This is probably due to an anatomical variation where the posterior medullary segment, prior to the development of the tumor, is located posterior to the fourth ventricle and medial to the tonsil, rather than lateral to the fourth ventricle and anterior to the tonsil.[2]

Fig. 7-1A,B. Fourth ventricle ependymoma. Right vertebral angiogram, arterial phase, lateral and frontal projections: same case as Figs. 7-2, 7-3A,B. The basilar artery (unlabeled arrows) is displaced anteriorly. The posterior medullary segment (3) of PICA is posteriorly displaced. The retrotonsillar segment (5) and the copular point (c) are posteriorly displaced. The superior vermian branch (s) of the superior cerebellar artery is also posteriorly displaced and stretched. On the frontal projection, the posterior medullary segment (3) is slightly laterally displaced, but the retrotonsillar segment (5) is not displaced.

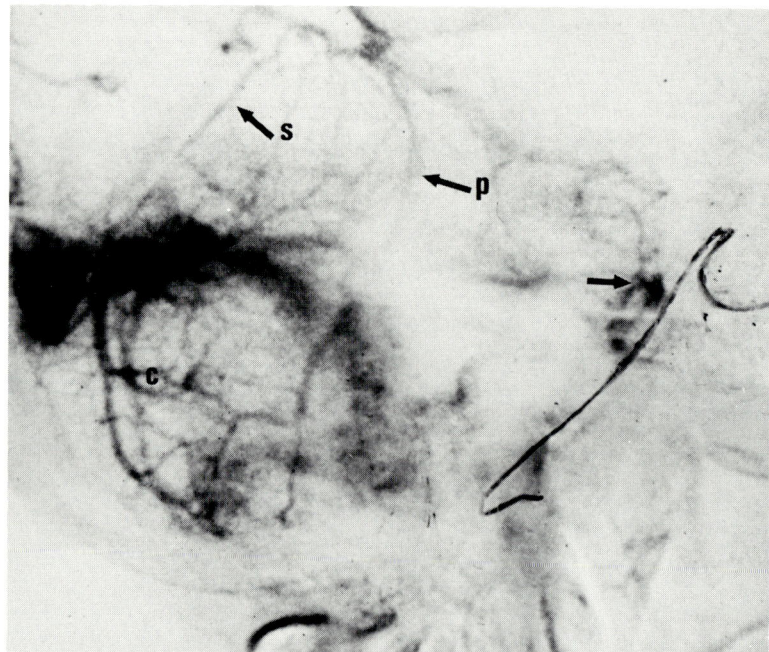

Fig. 7-2. Venous phase, lateral projection. Note the anterior displacement of the pontine segment of the ponto-mesencephalic vein (unlabeled arrow) and the posterior displacement of the precentral cerebellar vein (p). The venous copular point (c) and the superior vermian vein (s) are also posteriorly displaced.

Lateral Displacements

These are seen on the semiaxial projection. The major displacement involves the PICA (Fig. 7-13). The supratonsillar segment is stretched and laterally displaced. Seldom is this segment displaced and stretched in isolation, and often the posterior medullary and tonsillar segments form a single continuous curve which is convex laterally (Figs. 7-1B, 7-3B, 7-6B). In conjunction with a complementary convex lateral curve and stretching of the equivalent segments of the contralateral posterior inferior cerebellar artery, the appearances are indicative of a midline lesion.[6]

If the tumor compresses and invades the medulla, the lateral medullary segments are displaced laterally and can simulate a large pontine tumor (Fig. 7-4B).

Care must be taken not to overdiagnose enlargements of the fourth ventricle by noting only a laterally situated tonsillar segment on a semiaxial projection. This appearance is normal in those cases where the artery lies lateral

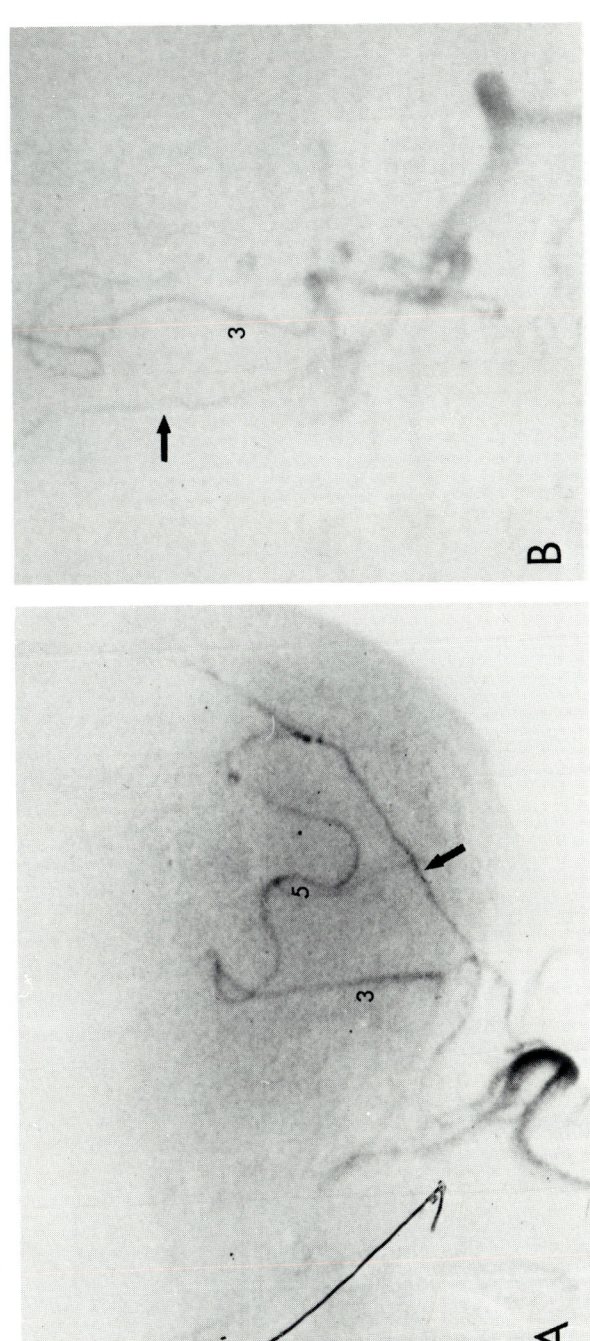

Fig. 7-3A,B. Left vertebral angiography, arterial phase, lateral and frontal projections. The posterior medullary segment (3) of the left PICA is stretched and slightly posteriorly displaced. It is also displaced to the left with a convex lateral curve. On the lateral projection, the posterior medullary segments of both PICAs place the mass in the midline. Note the prominent, but normal, posterior meningeal branch (arrow) of the vertebral artery.

to the tonsil (see Normal Variations, Chapter 4). Absence of associated supratentorial angiographic signs of hydrocephalus indicates that there is no obstruction of the fourth ventricle. With fourth ventricular enlargement, lateral displacement of the vein of the lateral recess of the fourth ventricle usually occurs (Figs. 7-5B, 7-7, 7-13). When ballooning of the fourth ventricle is marked, lateral displacement of the lateral anastomotic mesencephalic vein is also present.

Often with medulloblastomas, the tumors are present in both the fourth ventricle and the inferior vermis. In addition to the angiographic signs already described, stretching of the inferior vermian arteries and veins will be seen (Fig. 7-8). Takahashi and associates described enlargement of nodular branches of the inferior vermian artery as a sign of involvement of the vermis (Fig. 7-6A).[7] Involvement of the superior vermis will displace the precentral cerebellar vein anteriorly. The presence of tumor within the fourth ventricle may enlarge the choroidal branches of PICA.[8]

It is not uncommon for fourth ventricular tumors to grow out of the ventricle through the foramina. This feature can be seen with ependymomas, choroid plexus papillomas, and medulloblastomas.[1, 9-11] Extension may then occur posteriorly into the cisterna magna, laterally into the pontomedullary cistern, or anteriorly in front of the pons and cervical cord. When the tumor extends out of the fourth ventricle into the vallecula and cisterna magna, the copular point and inferior vermian artery and vein are elevated.[2, 5] The angiographic appearances can then be due to a combination of tumor mass in the fourth ventricle and tumor mass in the cisterna magna (see Figs. 7-4A, 7-5A, 7-6A). When the tumor extends into the cerebellopontine angle cistern, it may mimic a primary cerebellopontine angle tumor (Figs. 7-9A,B). With extracerebellar extensions, the differential diagnosis from a pontine glioma with exophytic extension may depend only on the position of the vein of the lateral recess of the fourth ventricle. The distinguishing feature is that with a fourth ventricular tumor, the vein is usually displaced laterally (Figs. 7-5B, 7-7, 7-13), whereas this is not an invariable feature of a pontine tumor since the tumor may involve the adjacent restiform body of the cerebellum (see Fig. 6-13).[2] Enlarged choroidal branches of PICA may be seen with fourth ventricle papillomas and meningiomas, and homogeneous stains may occur with fourth ventricle meningiomas (Fig. 7-5A).[12, 13]

More than with any other tumor group, the diagnosis of tumors within the fourth ventricle and their differentiation from pontine tumors requires high-quality angiograms with considerable vascular detail (see Table 6-1, p. 116). Pneumoencephalography and ventriculography should be obtained, however, when the diagnosis is in doubt, as often the vascular changes are too subtle or confusing to allow the diagnosis to be accurately made by angiography alone.

The differential diagnosis of fourth ventricular enlargement secondary to

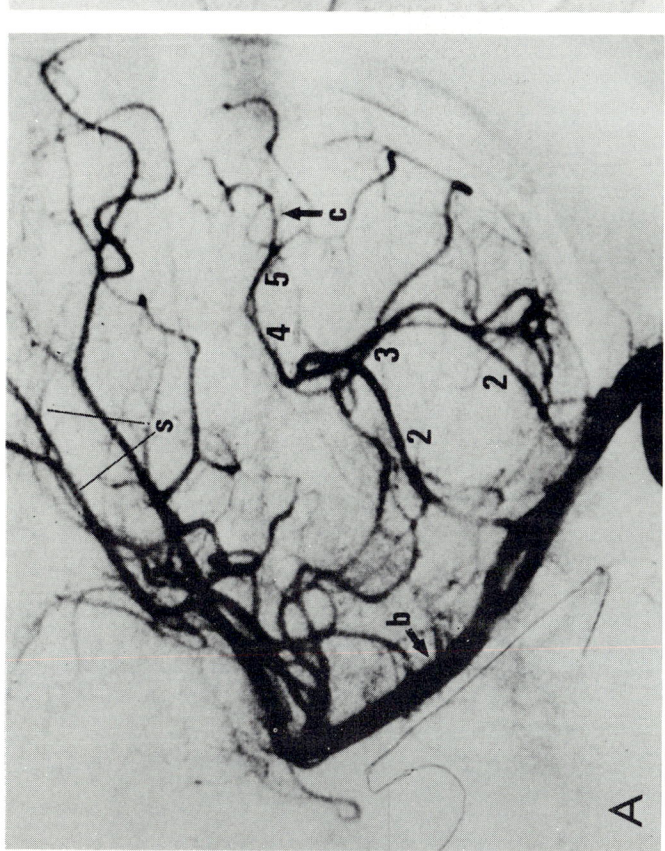
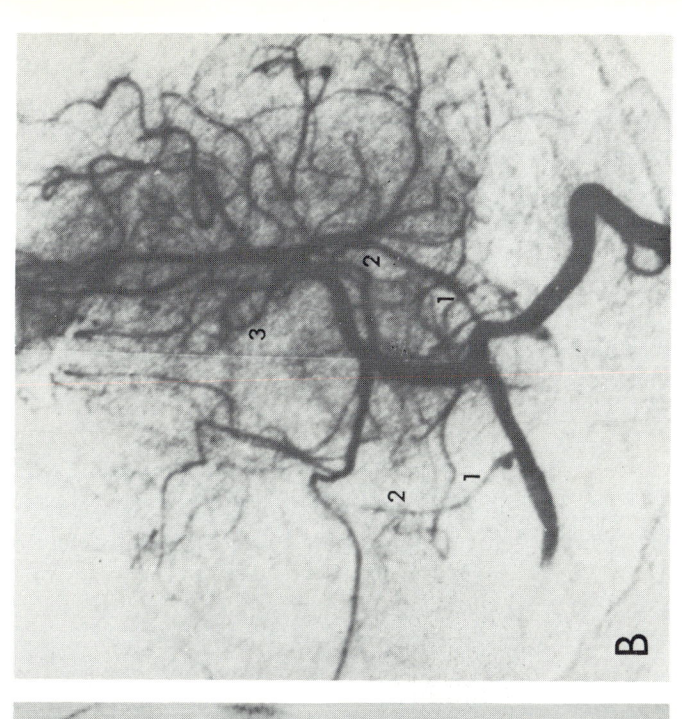

Fig. 7-4A,B. Fourth ventricle meningioma in a 3-year-old child. Left vertebral angiogram, arterial phase, lateral and frontal projections: same case as Fig. 7-5A,B. The basilar artery (b) is anteriorly displaced against the clivus. There is marked stretching of both lateral medullary segments (2) of PICA with posterior displacement of the left posterior medullary segment (3). The supratonsillar segment (4) is stretched. On the frontal projection, the anterior medullary segments (1) are stretched and laterally displaced. This is due to anterior compression with lateral expansion of the pons. The lateral (2) and posterior medullary (3) segments are also laterally displaced. On the lateral projection, the retrotonsillar segment (5) of the left PICA is posteriorly displaced. The copular point (c) is elevated indicating extension of the tumor into the cisterna magna. The superior vermian branches (s) of the superior cerebellar arteries are posterosuperiorly displaced.

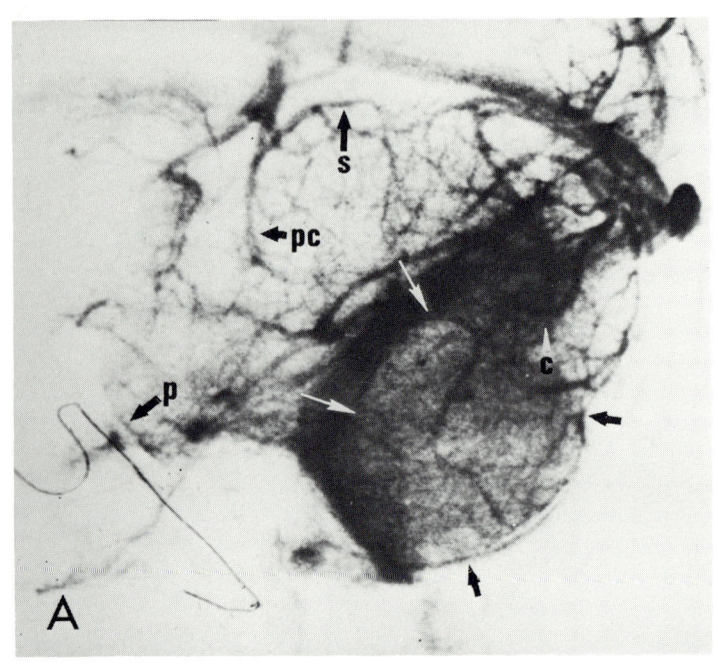

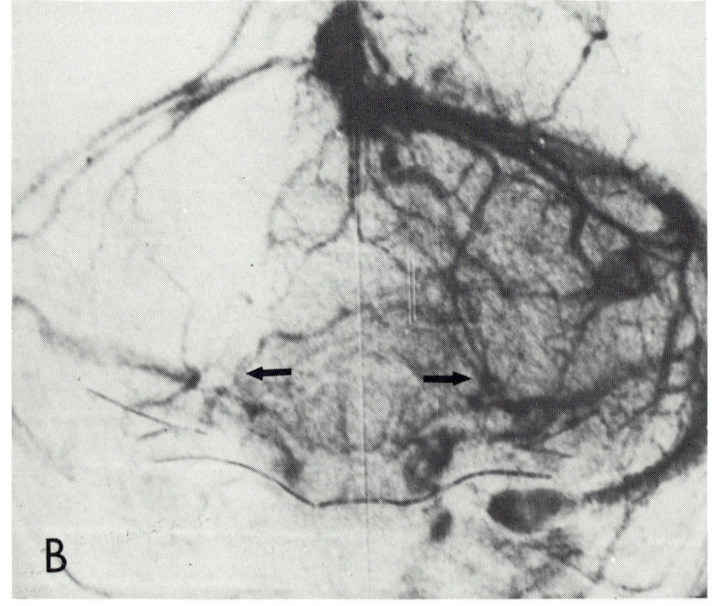

communicating hydrocephalus from enlargement due to a tumor may be difficult. Generally, the lateral sweep of the supratonsillar segment of PICA is less pronounced in communicating hydrocephalus (Fig. 7-10B). A useful differential point is that in communicating hydrocephalus, the basilar artery and ponto-mesencephalic vein are displaced away from the clivus because of the enlarged pontine and interpeduncular cisterns, whereas the artery and vein are compressed forward against the clivus in fourth ventricle tumors (Figs. 7-10A,B; 7-11, 7-12). Burns and co-workers, in 1972, considered that the angiographic changes of fourth ventricular enlargement secondary to hydrocephalus were indistinguishable from those of fourth ventricular enlargement secondary to tumor.[14] However, Huang and Wolf considered that the marked lateral bowing of the various segments of the PICA is absent in fourth ventricular enlargement secondary to hydrocephalus.[15]

REFERENCES

1. Koos WT, Miller MH: Intracranial Tumors of Infants and Children (ed 1). St. Louis, Mosby, 1971
2. Huang YP, Wolf BS: Angiographic features of brain stem tumors and differential diagnosis from fourth ventricle tumors. Am J Roentgenol 110:1, 1970
3. Huang YP, Wolf BS: Differential diagnosis of fourth ventricle tumors from brain stem tumors in angiography. Neuroradiology 1:4, 1970
4. Galligioni F, Bernardi R, Pellone M, Iraci G: The veins of the posterior cranial fossa: an angiographic study under pathologic conditions. Am J Roentgenol 110:39, 1970
5. Wilner HI, Navarro E, Bradley A, Eisenbrey B, Gracias V: The inferior vermian veins as a useful adjunct in the differentiation of brain stem tumors from midline cerebellar masses. Am J Roentgenol 108:605, 1973

Fig. 7-5A,B. Venous phase, lateral and frontal projections. The pontine segment of the ponto-mesencephalic vein (p) is anteriorly displaced. The precentral cerebellar vein (pc) is slightly anteriorly displaced with retention of its normal curvature. This indicates a mass effect behind the plane of the ventricle-aqueduct due to tumor in the cisterna magna. The superior vermian vein (s) is slightly elevated. The venous copular point (c) is elevated due to tumor mass in the cisterna magna. In the lateral projection, note the vascular stain (unlabeled arrows) of the meningioma. In the frontal projection, note the lateral displacement of the veins of the lateral recesses of the fourth ventricle (unlabeled arrows).

At postmortem, the tumor was seen to originate from the fourth ventricle, invade the pons, and extend into the cisterna magna.

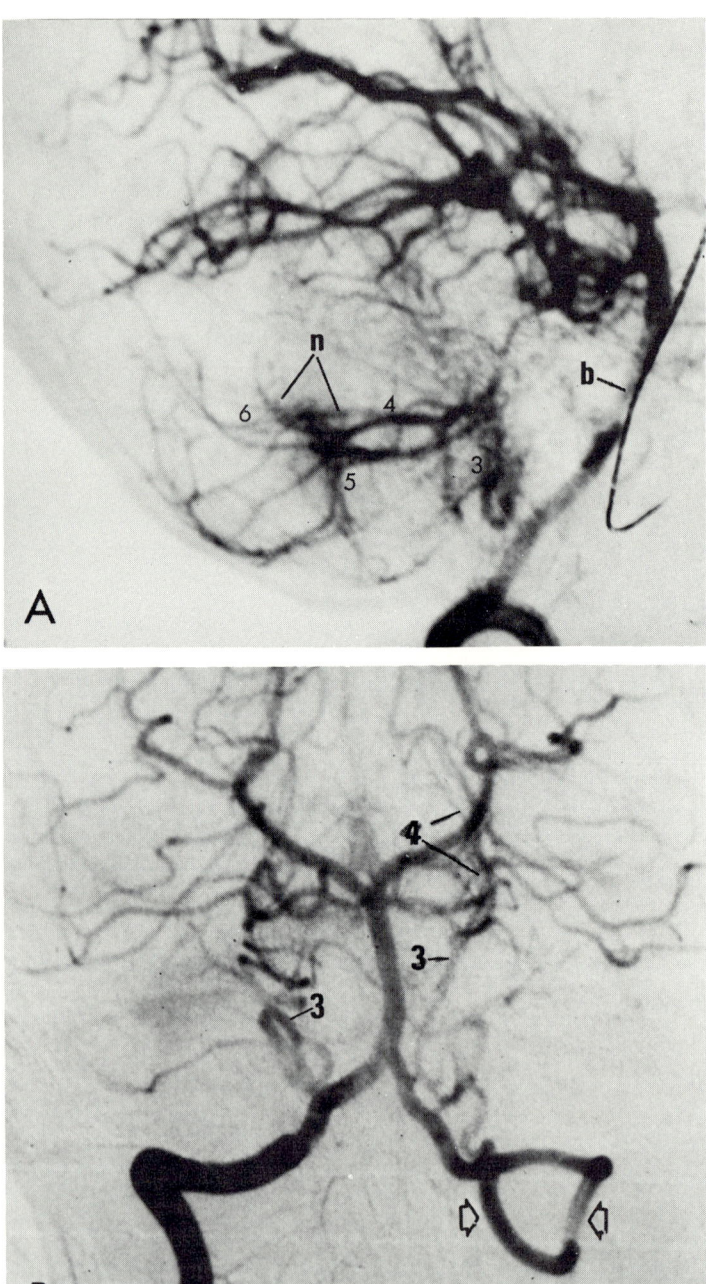

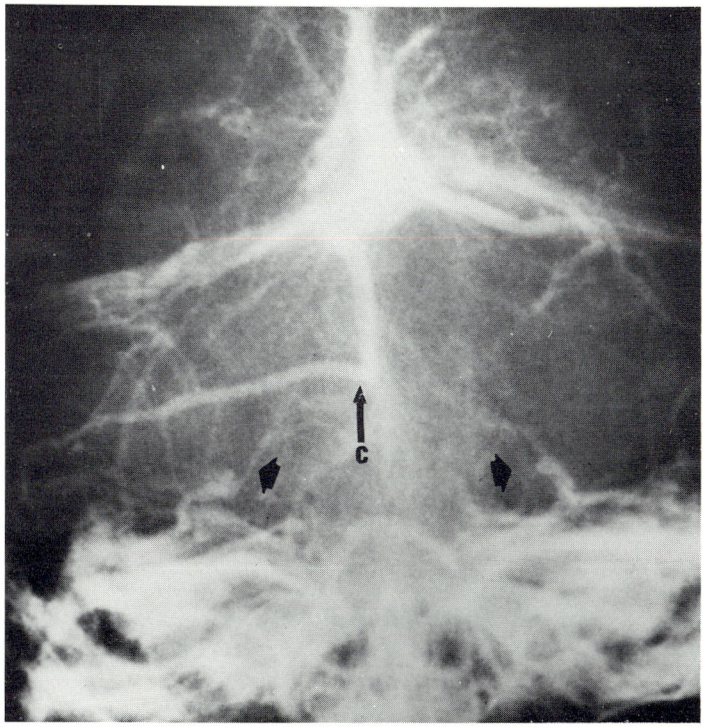

Fig. 7-7. Venous phase, frontal projection (non-subtracted film). There is an acute angulation at the junction of an inferior vermian vein and a left inferior hemispheric vein due to extension of the tumor into the cisterna magna and posterior displacement of the venous copular point (c). The veins of the lateral recesses are laterally displaced (arrows).

Fig. 7-6A,B. Medulloblastoma in a 6-year-old boy. Right vertebral angiogram, arterial phase, lateral and frontal projections: same case as Figs. 7.7, 7.8. The basilar artery (b) is anteriorly displaced. The posterior medullary segment (3) of PICA is anteriorly displaced, and on the frontal projection there is separation of the posterior medullary segments of the two PICAs. The supratonsillar segment (4) of the right PICA is stretched and laterally displaced, and the retrotonsillar segment (5) is posteriorly displaced. The inferior vermian branch (6) is elevated, indicating extension of the tumor into the cisterna magna. Note the nodular branch hypertrophy (n) with some tumor stain, which indicates involvement of the inferior vermis. The reflux of contrast material down the left vertebral artery is adequate to demonstrate a bifid vertebral artery (open arrows) which is a normal variant.

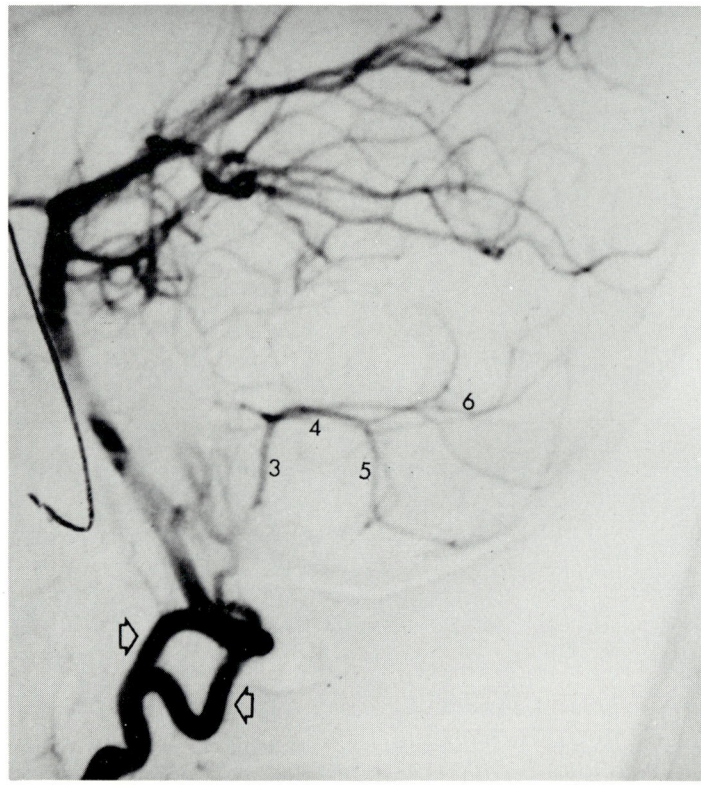

Fig. 7-8. Left vertebral angiogram, arterial phase, lateral projection. Note the bifid anomaly of the left vertebral artery (open arrows). The segments of PICA on the left side are displaced in an identical manner to that on the right side with anterior displacement of the posterior medullary segment (3), stretching of the supratonsillar segment (4), posterior displacement of the retrotonsillar segment (5), and stretching with elevation of the inferior vermian branch (6).

Fig. 7-9A,B. Ependymoma originating from the fourth ventricle with extension around the brainstem into the pontine and cerebellopontine angle cisterns. Right brachial angiogram, arterial phase, lateral and frontal projections (non-subtracted films). There is posterior displacement of the basilar artery (b) and superior and medial displacement of the anterior inferior cerebellar artery (a). (Courtesy of Am J Roentgenol 112:296, 1971.)

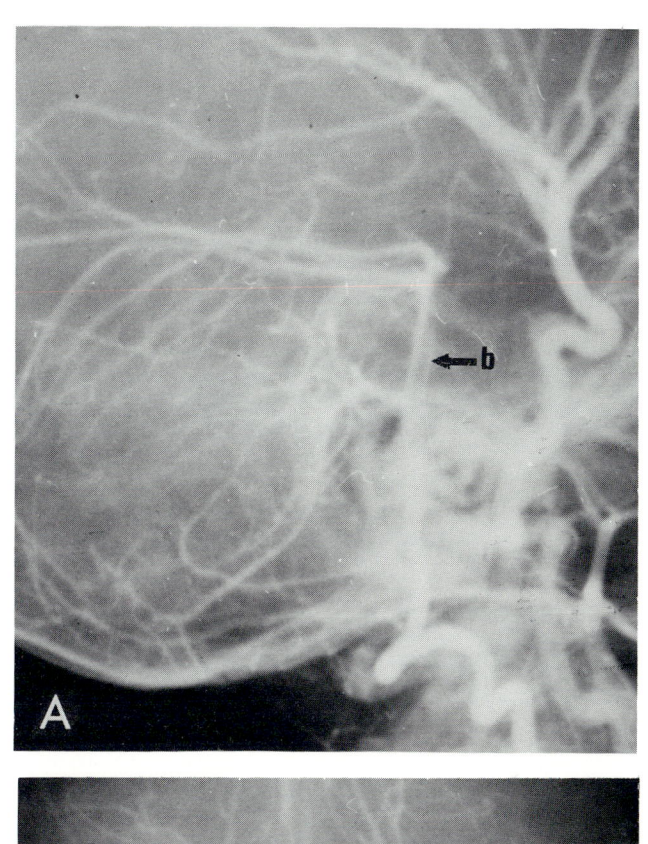

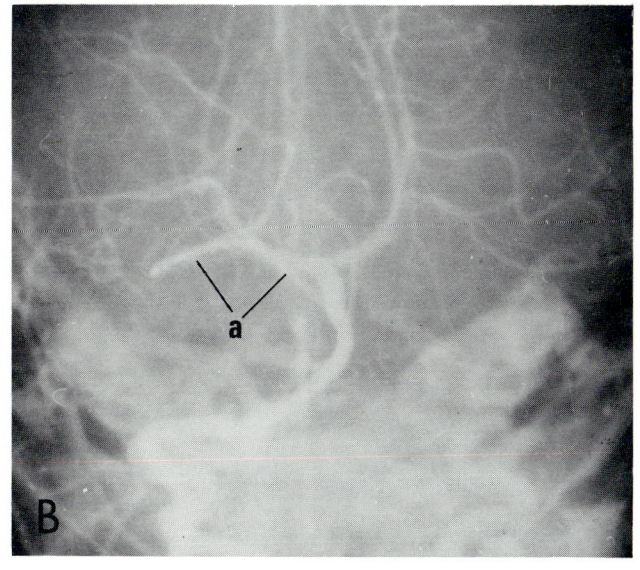

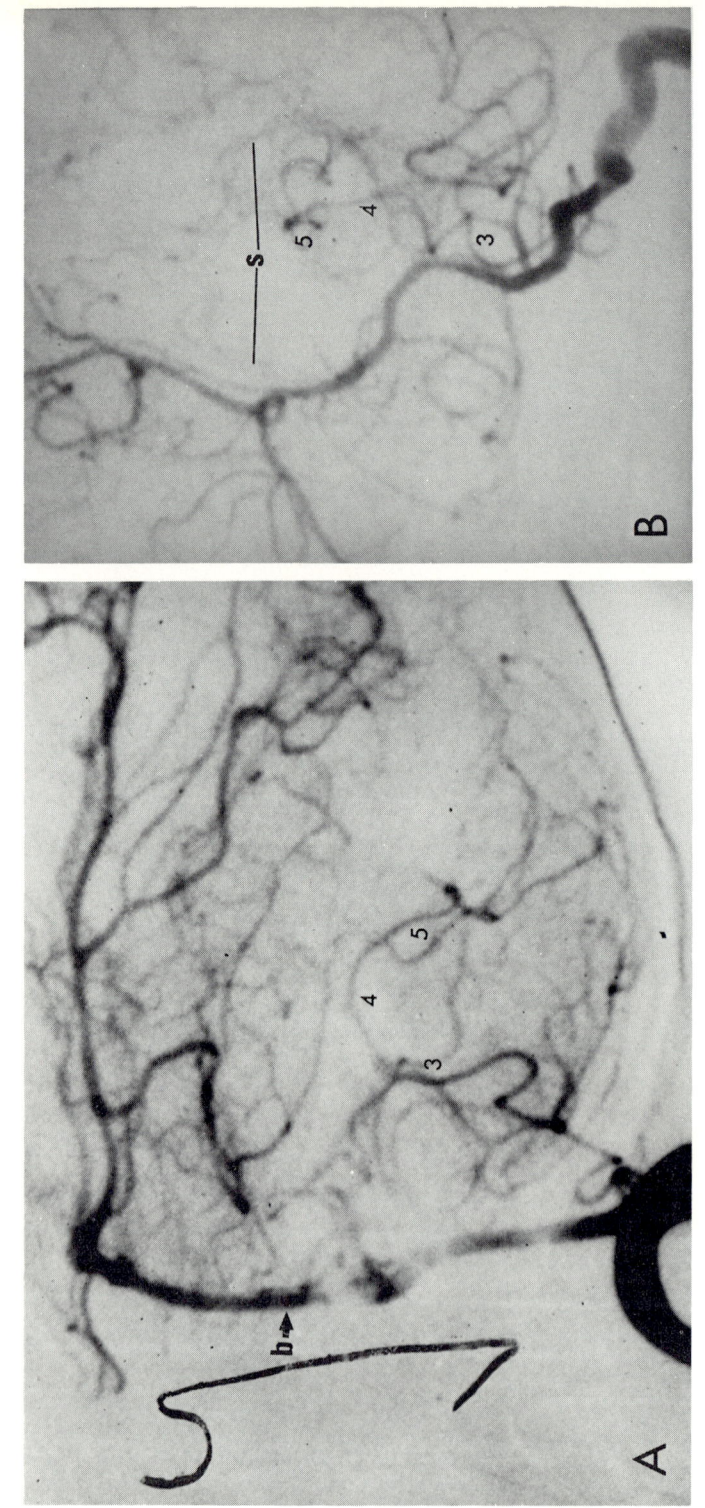

Fig. 7-10A,B. Communicating hydrocephalus. Left vertebral angiogram, arterial phase, lateral and frontal projections: same case as Figs. 7-11, 7-12. The basilar artery (b) is separated from the clivus. There is some lateral deviation of the supratonsillar segment (4) of PICA, but this is not pronounced. The superior cerebellar arteries (s) are moderately separated but relaxed. The posterior medullary (3) and retrotonsillar segment (5) of PICA are shown.

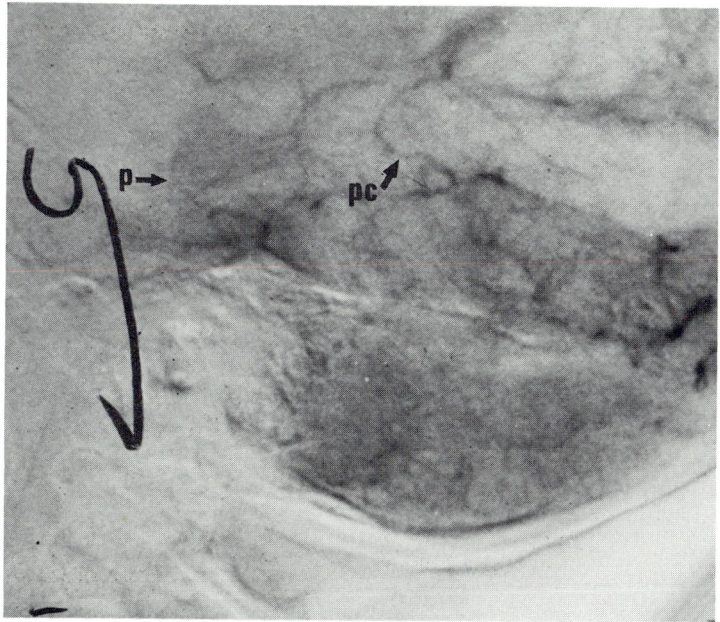

Fig. 7-11. Venous phase, lateral projection. The pontine vein (p) is separated from the clivus. The precentral cerebellar vein (pc) is elevated with a decrease in the collculo-central angle which is indicative of an enlarged fourth ventricle.

6. Peeters FL: The vertebral angiogram in patients with tumours in or near the midline. Neuroradiology 5:53, 1973
7. Takahashi M, Okudera T, Fukui M, Kitamura K: The choroidal and nodular branches of the posterior inferior cerebellar artery. Their value in the diagnosis of medulloblastomas. Radiology 103:347, 1972
8. Takahashi M: Atlas of Vertebral Angiography. Tokyo, Igaku Shoin, Ltd, 1974
9. Russel DS, Rubinstein LJ: Pathology of Tumours of the Nervous System (ed 2). London, Arnold, 1963
10. Epstein BS, Epstein JA, Carras R: Extension of posterior fossa tumors, particularly intraventricular fourth ventricle tumors, into the upper cervical spinal canal. Am J Roentgenol 110:31, 1970
11. Wickbom I, Hanafee W: Soft tissue masses immediately below the foramen magnum. Acta Radiol [Diagn] (Stockh) 1:647, 1963
12. Rodriguez-Carbajal J, Palacios E: Intraventricular meningiomas of the fourth ventricle. Am J Roentgenol 120:27, 1974

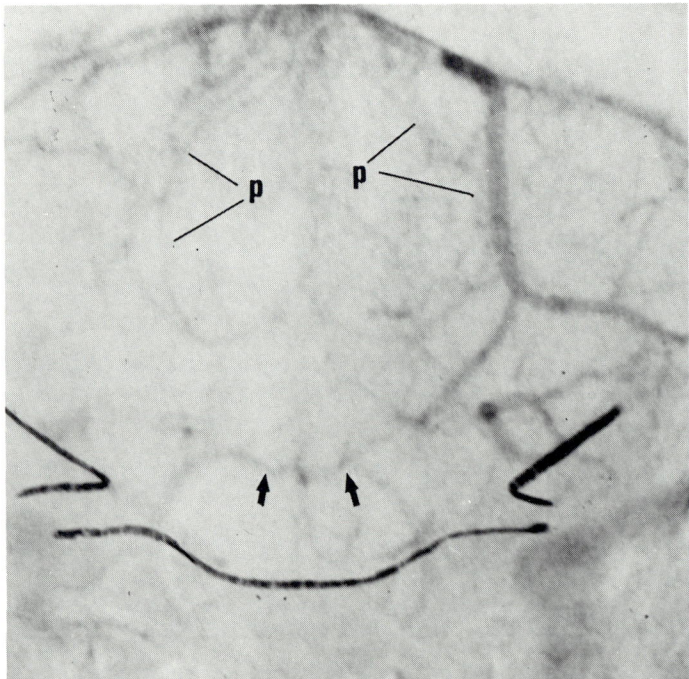

Fig. 7-12. Venous phase, frontal projection. The transverse pontine vein (arrows) is separated from the clivus. There is an increase in the sweep of the posterior mesencephalic veins (p) as they encircle the midbrain.

13. Hoffman JC, Bufkin WJ, Richardson HD: Primary intraventricular meningiomas of the fourth ventricle. Am J Roentgenol 115:100, 1972
14. Burns JB, Hoffman JC, Brylski JR: Posterior inferior cerebellar artery in fourth ventricular dilatation. Acta Radiol [Diagn] (Stockh) 13:58, 1972
15. Huang YP, Wolf BS: Angiographic features of fourth ventricle tumors with special reference to the posterior inferior cerebellar artery. Am J Roentgenol 107:543, 1969

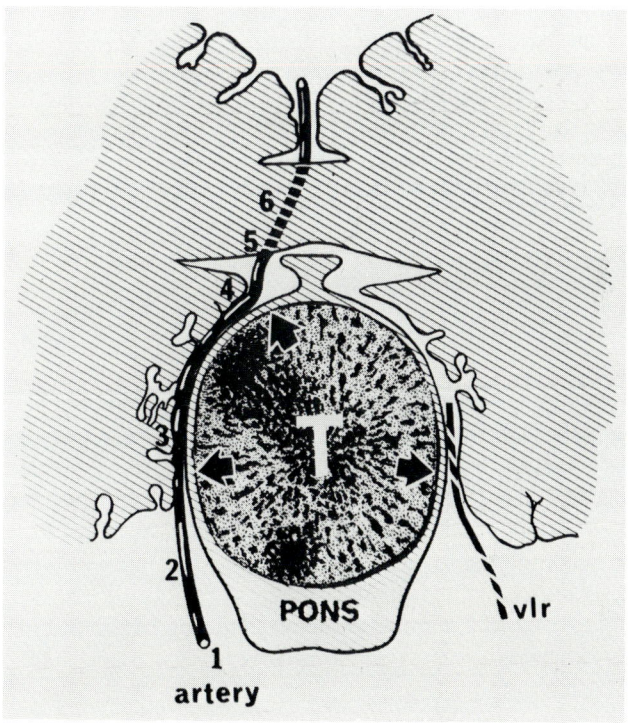

Fig. 7-13. Line diagram of fourth ventricle tumor demonstrating lateral displacement of lateral medullary (2) and posterior medullary (3) segments and posterolateral displacement of the supratonsillar (4) and retrotonsillar (5) segments. The vein of the lateral recess (vlr) is laterally displaced. (Compare with Fig. 6-13.)

8
Vermian and Hemispheric Tumors (Plates VI and VII*)

Frequently, tumors of the midline vermis infiltrate the lateral cerebellar hemispheres and vice versa. Vermian and hemispheric tumors will therefore be considered together. In children, medulloblastomas and cystic astrocytomas are the most common tumors found in this region. In adults, the most common tumors are most often metastatic. The source of the metastases includes the lung, gastrointestinal tract, kidney, and breast. The most common primary tumors in adults are the hemangioblastomas.

Radiologically, the vermis and hemisphere can be divided into inferior and superior divisions.

INFERIOR VERMIAN AND INFERIOR HEMISPHERIC TUMORS

When a tumor involves the inferior vermis, the basilar artery and pontomesencephalic vein often are anteriorly displaced. This is a nonspecific appearance and is present with any space-occupying mass in the cerebellum. The fourth ventricle is anteriorly displaced, and this is evident both by anterior displacement of the choroidal point and by compression of the supratonsillar segment of the posterior inferior cerebellar artery (Figs. 8-1A, 8-2, 8-3A). The retrotonsillar segment of the posterior inferior cerebellar artery is anteriorly displaced.[1] The copular points of both the inferior vermian artery and the inferior vermian vein are displaced inferiorly and posteriorly and, accordingly,

*See color plates, page 34.

on a lateral film lie close to the inner table of the skull (Figs. 8-2, 8-4A, 8-4B).[2-5]

On a semiaxial projection, the midline position of the inferior vermian artery and vein indicates the midline position of the tumor (Figs. 8-1B, 8-3B, 8-4B). It is possible, however, for the inferior vermian veins, lying in sulci on either side of the inferior vermis, to be separated when the tumor is in the vermis.[5]

When the tumor involves the inferior cerebellar hemisphere, there is both anterior and lateral displacement of the fourth ventricle. This has an effect on the branches of the posterior inferior cerebellar artery and can best be appreciated on the semiaxial projection. The choroid arch, which normally can lie up to 5 mm from the midline, is displaced contralaterally across the midline, away from the side of the tumor (Fig. 8-5). On the normal side, the choroid arch is displaced ipsilaterally. The supratonsillar segments of the posterior inferior cerebellar arteries are similarly displaced. It is important to define the choroid arches and the supratonsillar segments on both sides. If only the artery on the normal side is seen, the ipsilateral displacement could indicate either a fourth ventricular tumor or a hemispheric tumor. Opacification of the artery on the abnormal side helps to differentiate between the two possibilities.

The vein of the lateral recess of the fourth ventricle is displaced medially away from the tumor (Fig. 8-6).

Major displacements are seen in the inferior hemispheric and vermian branches of the posterior inferior cerebellar artery and in the inferior hemispheric and vermian veins. The hemispheric branches of the posterior inferior cerebellar artery are stretched around the neoplasm (Figs. 8-7, 8-9, 8-15). Inferior hemispheric veins are stretched (Figs. 8-6, 8-10). The inferior vermian artery is displaced away from the tumor.[2,3,6-8] This can be well appreciated on a semiaxial projection (Fig. 8-5). The inferior vermian vein is similarly displaced. On occasion, venous filling on the side of a tumor is poor due to venous compression by the tumor. This sign is valuable, however, only if there is good arterial opacification on the side of the tumor.[9,10]

Takahashi and associates described hypertrophy and posterior displacement of the nodular branches of the posterior inferior cerebellar artery when medulloblastomas involve the nodulus.[11,12] These vessels, which are not usually seen unless pathologically enlarged, originate from the supratonsillar segment of the posterior inferior cerebellar artery (see Fig. 7-6A).

Cerebellar Tonsil Tumor

When the cerebellar tonsil is involved by tumor, characteristic changes appear on the angiogram. Vessels lying in front of the tonsil are displaced anteriorly, vessels behind the tonsil posteriorly, and vessels medial to the tonsil

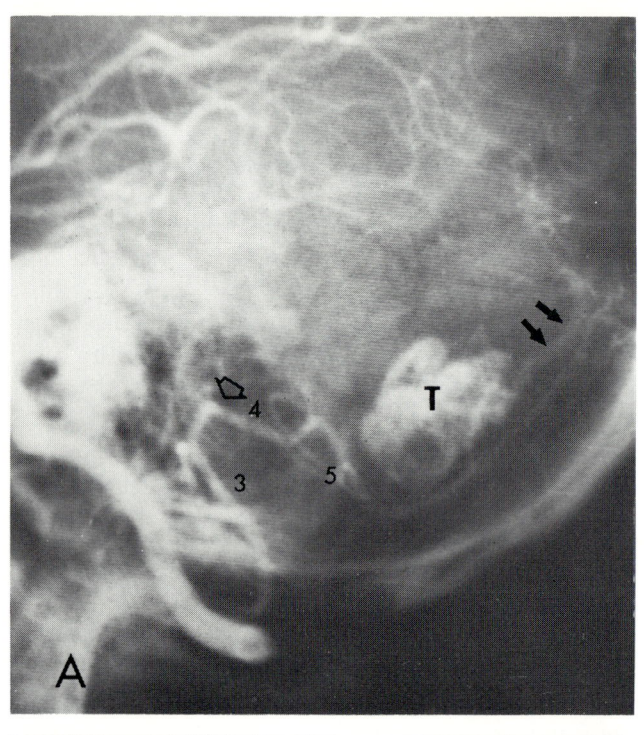

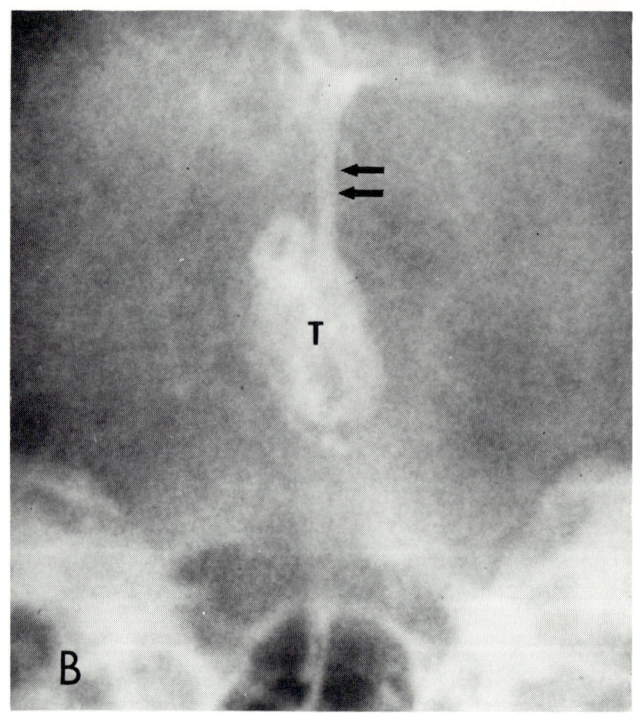

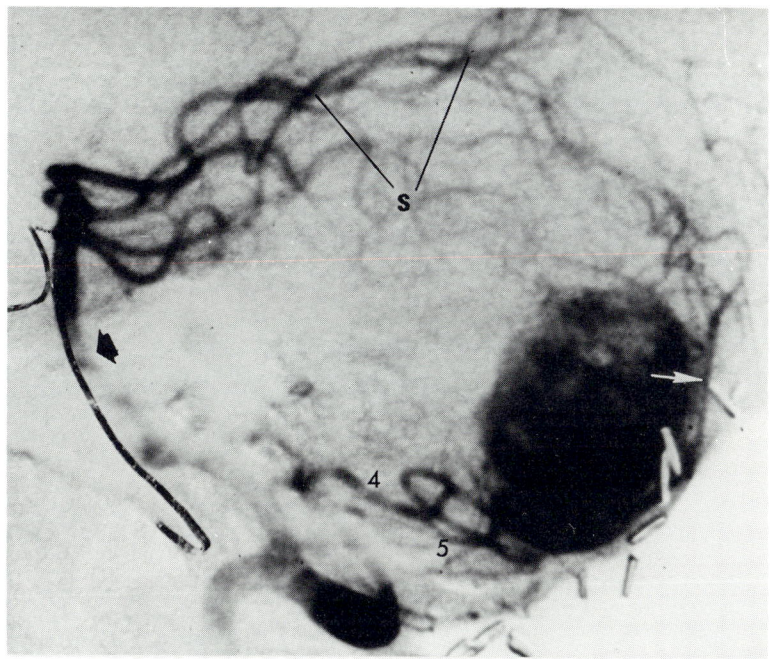

Fig. 8-2. Same patient as Fig. 8-1 after surgery and tumor recurrence; left vertebral angiogram, arterial phase, lateral projection. The basilar artery (black arrow) is displaced anteriorly against the clivus. There is now marked anterior displacement and flattening of the supratonsillar (4) and retrotonsillar (5) segments of PICA. The large tumor nodule has displaced the inferior vermian artery (white arrow) against the inner table of the skull. There is also upward displacement of the quadrigeminal and supraculminate segments and the superior vermian branch (s) of the superior cerebellar artery, which indicates involvement of the superior vermis.

contralaterally. Due to the many variations possible in the distribution of the branches of the posterior inferior cerebellar artery, displacements may be difficult to appreciate. Classically, on the lateral projection, the posterior medullary segment is displaced anteriorly, the supratonsillar segment is stretched, and the retrotonsillar segment is displaced posteriorly. The tonsil-

---

Fig. 8-1A,B. Inferior vermian hemangioblastoma. Left vertebral angiogram, arterial lateral and venous frontal projections (non-subtracted films). There is slight anterior displacement of the posterior medullary segment (3) of PICA and of the chorodial point (open arrow) with downward displacement of the supratonsillar segment (4). The retrotonsillar segment (5) is also anteriorly displaced. A vascular tumor nodule (T) is seen, with an early draining inferior vermian vein (paired arrows). (Courtesy Am J Roentgenol 110:56, 1970.)

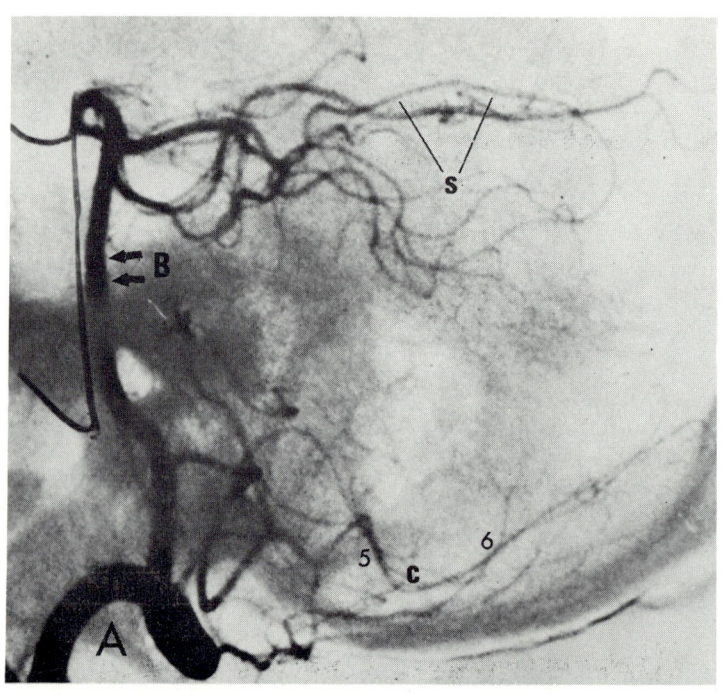
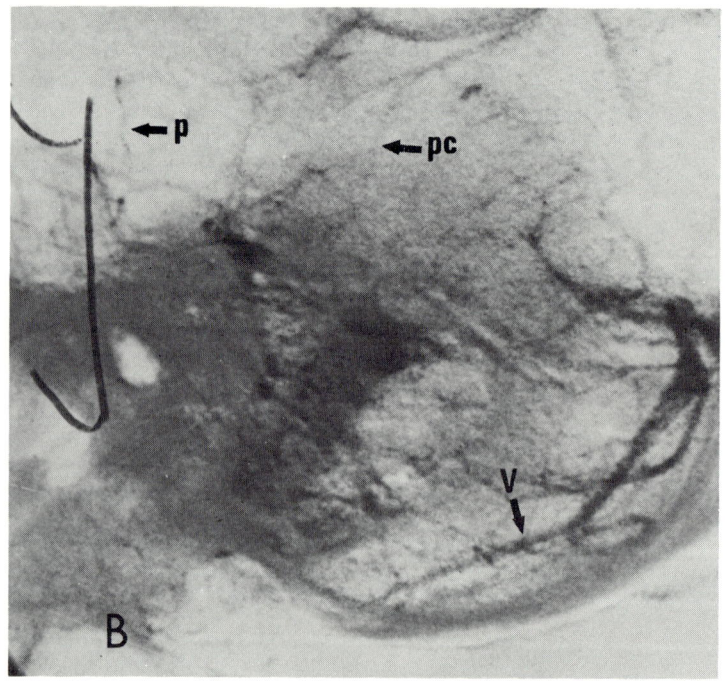

lohemispheric branch may be stretched around the tumor (Fig. 8-11). On the semiaxial projection, the supratonsillar segment is displaced contralaterally across the midline.[1]

TONSILLAR HERNIATION

Cerebellar tumors may be associated with herniation of the cerebellar tonsils through the foramen magnum. Compression of the medulla oblongata by the impacted tonsils may be fatal to the patient.[13]

Extension of the caudal loop (lateral medullary segment) of the posterior inferior cerebellar artery below the foramen magnum is not a reliable sign of tonsillar herniation since the caudal loop may normally lie up to 20 mm below the foramen magnum (Fig. 4-12).[14] Extension of the tonsillar branches of the tonsillohemispheric artery below the foramen magnum, however, has been described in the Arnold-Chiari malformation and referred to in cases of tonsillar herniation.[2] This sign is best seen on a lateral projection (Fig. 8-9). It is possible, however, for the tonsils to herniate through the foramen magnum without involving the tonsillar branches if the branches do not lie over the pole of the tonsil. Margolis and Newton considered that with tonsillar herniation, the hemispheric branches of the posterior inferior cerebellar artery are stretched and herniate through the foramen magnum.[15] This can best be appreciated on the anteroposterior film with the central ray 5° cephalad to the canthomeatal line (modified Caldwell projection). With this projection, the plane of the foramen magnum is viewed tangentially (Fig. 8-8).

Tonsillar herniation can also be diagnosed if the inferior retrotonsillar branch of the inferior vermian vein is seen below the plane of the foramen magnum (Fig. 8-12A,B). The differentiation of tonsillar herniation due to the Arnold-Chiari malformation from that due to a tumor may be difficult to appreciate unless there are other signs of a tumor mass present.

Fig. 8-3A,B. Vermian cystic astrocytoma. Left vertebral angiogram, arterial and venous phases, lateral projections: same case as Fig. 8-4A,B. The basilar artery (B) is displaced anteriorly against the clivus. The retrontonsillar segment (5) and the inferior vermian branch (6) of PICA are displaced inferiorly. The copular point (c) is depressed. Elevation of the quadrigeminal and supraculminate segments and the superior vermian branch (s) of the superior cerebellar artery indicates involvement of most of the midline vermis. The pontine segment (p) of the ponto-mesencephalic vein is displaced anteriorly, while the inferior vermian vein (V) is displaced inferiorly. The precentral cerebellar vein (pc) is stretched and displaced anteriorly.

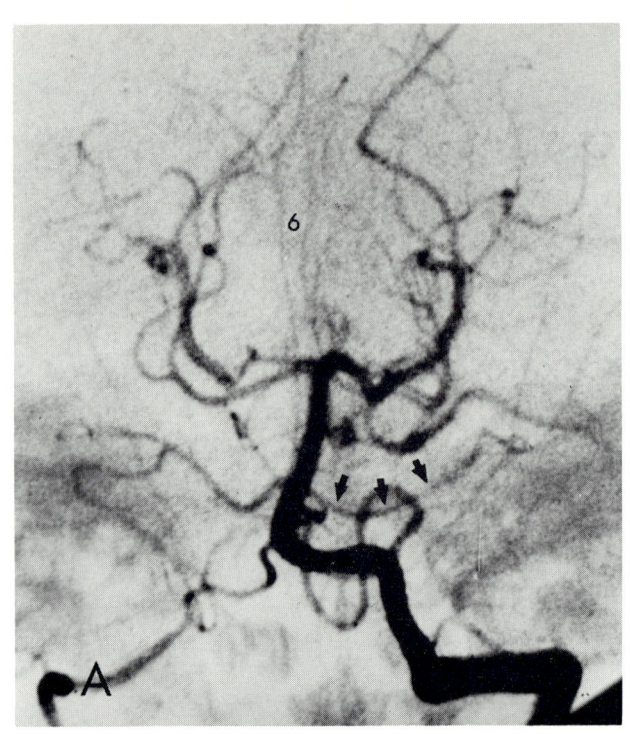

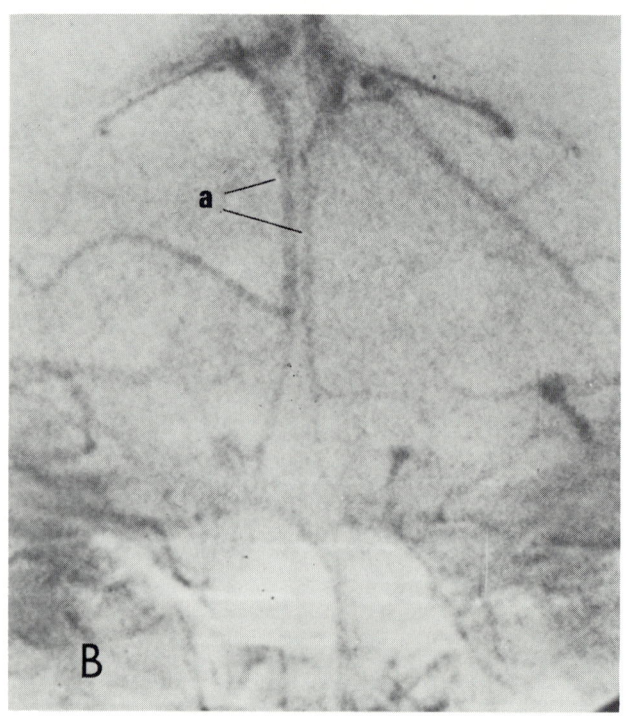

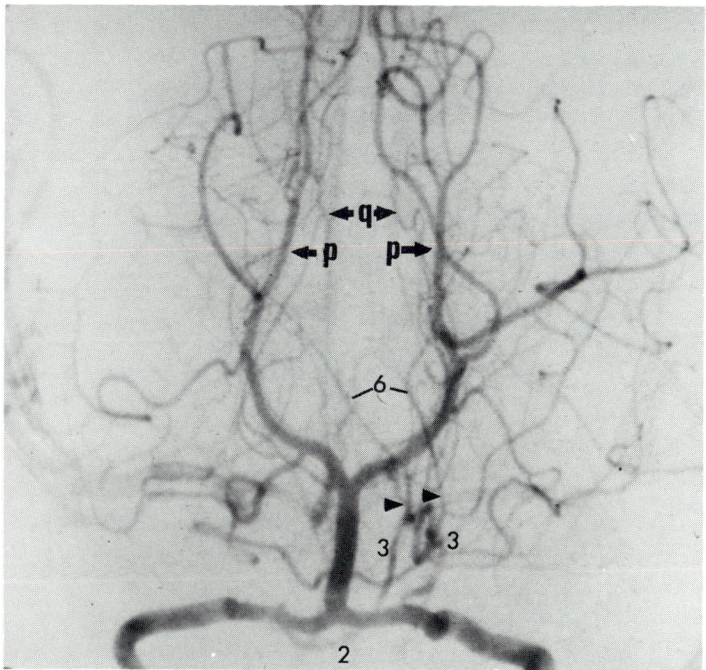

Fig. 8-5. Right inferior hemispheric astrocytoma. Left vertebral angiogram, arterial phase, frontal projection. (Note reflux down right vertebral artery. Same case as Figs. 8-6 through 8-10.) The posterior medullary segments (3) of both PICAs are displaced across the midline and to the left. The major displacement involves the choroid arches (arrowheads) and adjacent segments that are also displaced across the midline. The inferior vermian branches (6) are stretched but gradually return to the midline. The quadrigeminal segments of the posterior cerebral (p) and of the superior cerebellar (q) arteries are separated.

SUPERIOR VERMIAN AND SUPERIOR HEMISPHERIC TUMORS

With tumors in the superior vermis and superior hemisphere, the fourth ventricle and upper aqueduct are displaced anteriorly. As a result of the anterior displacement of the brainstem, there is anterior displacement of

---

Fig. 8-4A,B. Left vertebral angiogram, arterial and venous phases, frontal projections. The left anterior inferior cerebellar artery (arrows) is displaced downward and anteriorly, indicating some involvement of the left hemisphere. The inferior vermian branches (6) of PICA and the inferior vermian veins (a) are in the midline, which indicates the midline vermian involvement.

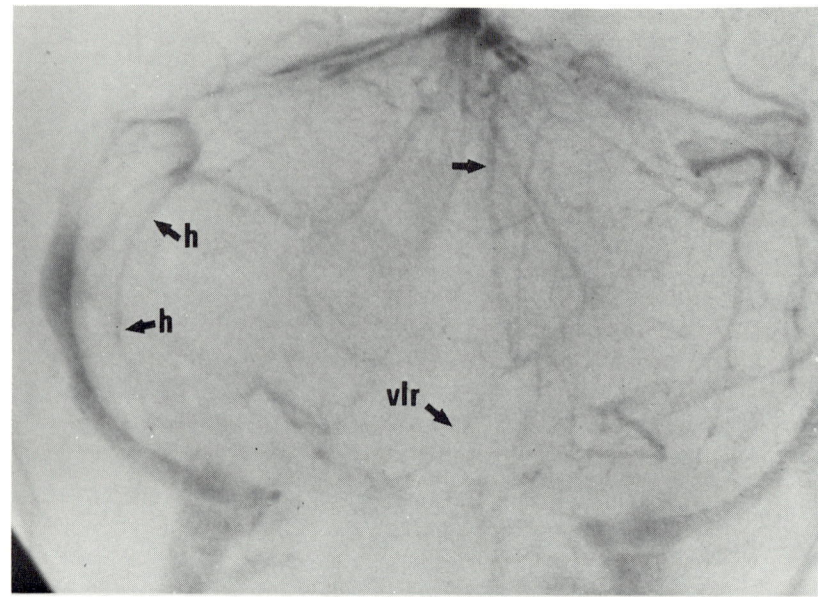

Fig. 8-6. Venous phase, frontal projection. The vein of the right lateral recess (vlr) of the fourth ventricle is displaced to the left. Inferior hemispheric veins (h) are displaced laterally and stretched. An inferior vermian vein (unlabeled arrow) lies to the left of the midline. The significance of this appearance is uncertain, however, as the vein need not normally lie in the midline.

the basilar artery and ponto-mesencephalic vein. The supraculminate and superior vermian branches of the superior cerebellar arteries are stretched and displaced upward (Figs. 8-13, 8-18). The precentral cerebellar vein is anteriorly displaced (Figs. 8-14, 8-19, 8-22).[4, 16, 19] The superior vermian vein is also displaced superiorly, obliterating the space between the vein and the straight sinus (Figs. 8-19, 8-22). If the tumor is sufficiently large, there is downward displacement of the choroidal loop and inferior vermian branches of the posterior inferior cerebellar artery. There is also downward displacement of the inferior vermian vein.

When the tumor involves the superior cerebellar hemisphere rather than the superior vermis, the major angiographic effect is on the marginal and hemispheric branches of the superior cerebellar artery (Figs. 8-16, 8-21). [4, 6, 7, 17, 18] If the tumor involves the anterior and lateral aspects of the cerebellum, the marginal branch is stretched (Fig. 8-21). If the lesion involves the superior aspect of the cerebellum, the hemispheric branches of the superior cerebellar artery are stretched. On the lateral projection, differentiation between the marginal and hemispheric branches of the two sides cannot be made.

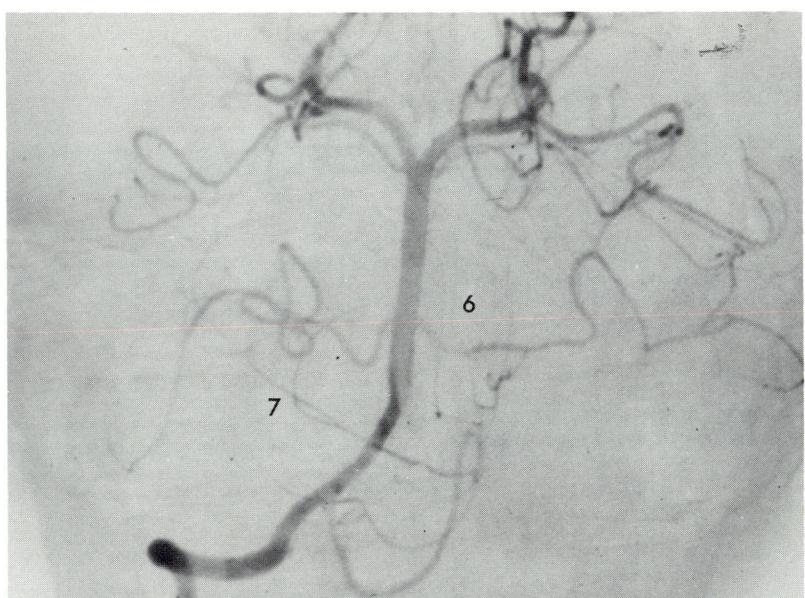

Fig. 8-7. Right vertebral angiogram, arterial phase, modified Caldwell projection. This projection in which the basilar artery is seen en face separates out the posterior inferior, anterior inferior, and superior cerebellar arteries. The displacement of the inferior vermian branches (6) of PICA is well seen. Note also the stretching of the hemispheric branches (7) of PICA.

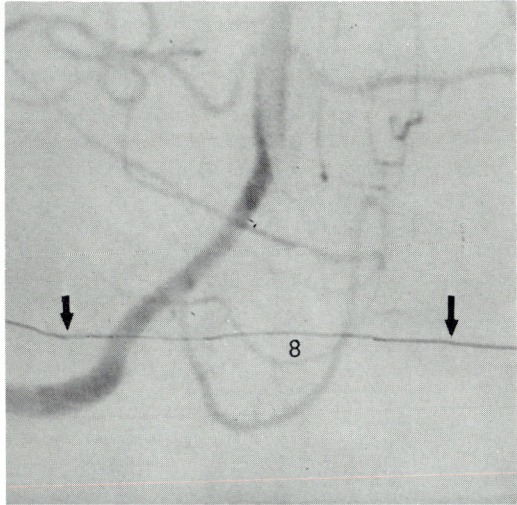

Fig. 8-8. Close-up view of Fig. 8-7. The tonsillohemispheric branch (8) of the posterior inferior cerebellar artery is below the plane of the foramen magnum (arrows), indicating tonsillar herniation.

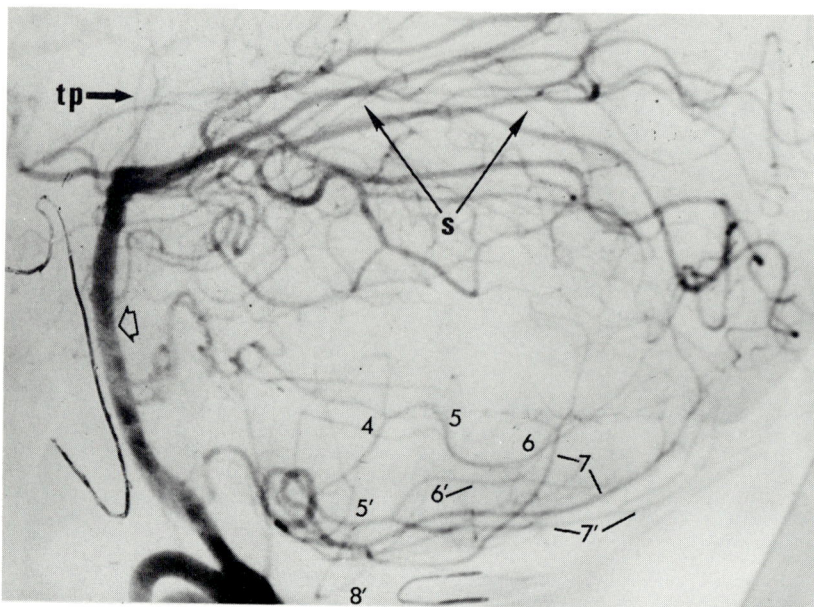

Fig. 8-9. Left vertebral angiogram, arterial phase, lateral projection. The basilar artery (open arrow) is displaced anteriorly against the clivus. The supratonsillar (4), retrotonsillar (5), and inferior vermian (6) branches of the left posterior inferior cerebellar artery are in a relatively normal position. The equivalent segments (5′, 6′) of the right posterior inferior cerebellar artery are displaced inferiorly and stretched. The hemispheric branches of both the left (7) and right (7′) posterior inferior cerebellar arteries are stretched with the right hemispheric branches closely applied to the inner table of the skull. The right tonsillohemispheric branch (8′) is displaced below the plane of the foramen magnum. The quadrigeminal and supraculminate segments together with the superior vermian branch (s) of the superior cerebellar artery are stretched and displaced superiorly. These angiographic appearances suggest that while the bulk of the tumor lies in the right inferior hemisphere, it is large enough to involve the superior hemisphere. The thalamoperforate arteries (tp) are stretched, indicating third ventricle dilatation secondary to an obstructive hydrocephalus.

A semiaxial projection, however, identifies the side of the mass lesion. A large hemispheric lesion will cause lateral displacement and stretching of PICA and its branches (Fig. 8-15).

Stretching of the superior hemispheric veins around the tumor also occurs with superior hemispheric mass lesions (Figs. 8-17, 8-19).[19] Flattening of the brachial vein indicates pressure on the brachial peduncle by an adjacent tumor (Fig. 8-20).

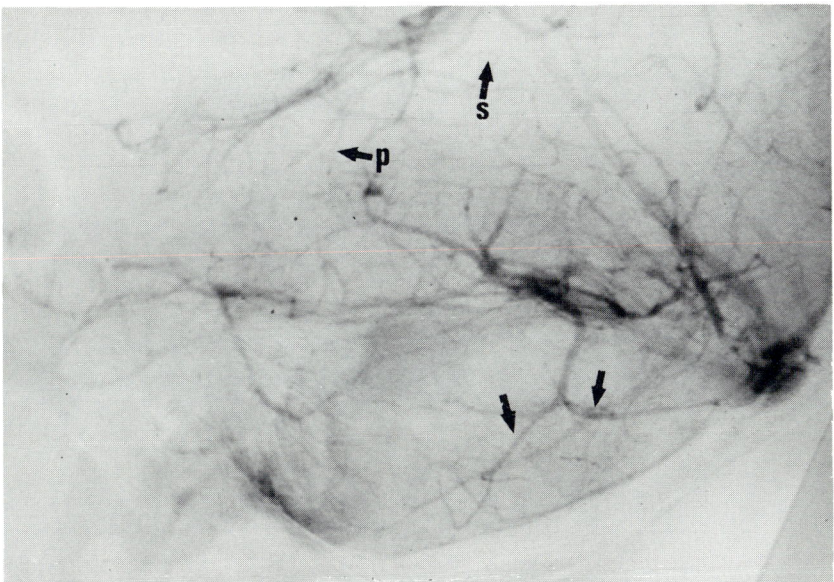

Fig. 8-10. Venous phase, lateral projection. Inferior hemispheric veins are stretched (arrows). The precentral cerebellar vein (p) is anteriorly displaced. The superior vermian vein (s) is displaced superiorly.

On occasion, a tumor may compress all the hemispheric veins and prevent them from filling.

When a tumor of the cerebellum is large and in the midline, upward herniation of the vermis through the tentorial notch can occur.[20] This causes separation of the quadrigeminal segments of the posterior cerebral artery (Fig. 8-21). The appearances on the semiaxial projection can simulate an intra-axial brainstem tumor. The position of the precentral cerebellar vein will correctly indicate the location of the tumor. In a brainstem tumor, the vein is displaced posteriorly; in a vermian tumor, the vein is displaced anteriorly (Figs. 8-14, 8-22, 6-2). Furthermore, there is upward displacement of the superior cerebellar arterial branches in vermian tumors, and lateral displacement in superior hemispheric tumors (Figs. 8-3A, 8-21). These displacements do not occur with pontine tumors unless there are exophytic components of the tumor displacing the hemispheric branches. Separation of the posterior cerebral and superior cerebellar arteries can also be seen in extra-axial midline tentorial edge tumors (see next paragraph).

With extra-axial tumors originating from the leaf of the tentorium, such as

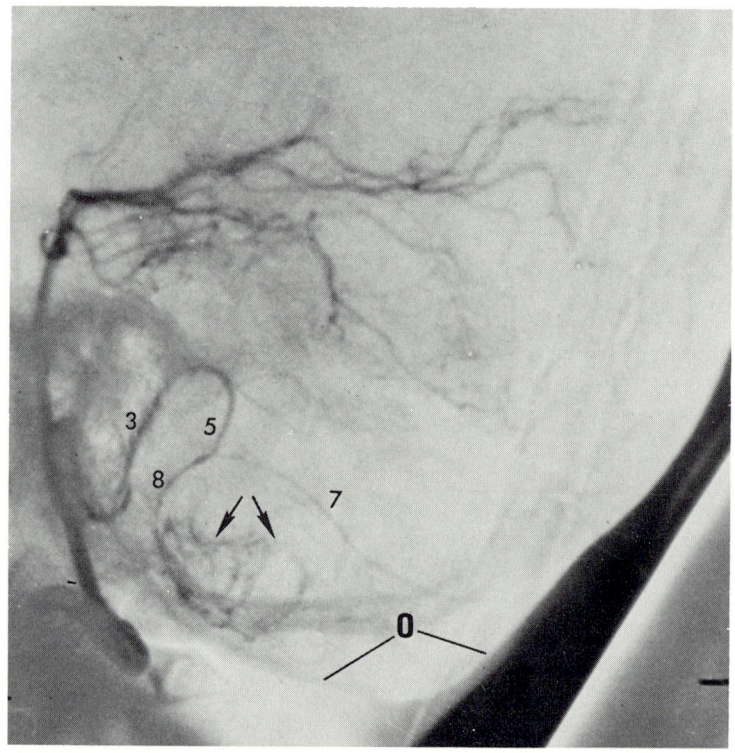

Fig. 8-11. Oligodendroglioma of the cerebellar tonsil and inferior cerebellar hemisphere. Left vertebral angiogram, arterial phase, lateral projection. The posterior medullary segment (3) of the left posterior inferior cerebellar artery is displaced anteriorly, and there is marked anterior bowing of the tonsillohemispheric branch (8). The retrotonsillar segment (5) is indicated. The hemispheric branch (7) is stretched, indicating extension of the tumor into the inferior cerebellar hemisphere. Note the tumor vessels (arrows) and the asymmetrical bulging of the occipital squamosa (O). This latter sign indicates a chronic expanding process in a young patient's skull when the bone is moderately malleable. (Courtesy of Am J Roentgenol 112:296, 1971.)

Fig. 8-12A,B. Cerebellar hemispheric hemangioblastoma. Left vertebral angiogram, venous phase, frontal and lateral projections. Note the vascular stain (T) with scattered central radiolucencies characteristic of a hemangioblastoma. The inferior retrotonsillar branch (arrows) of the inferior vermian vein is displaced downward and medially. On the frontal view, the vein may be confused with a medially displaced vein of the lateral recess of the fourth ventricle. It would be unlikely, however, for the vein of the lateral recess to lie below the plane of the foramen magnum. At surgery, tumor extended into the cerebellar tonsil.

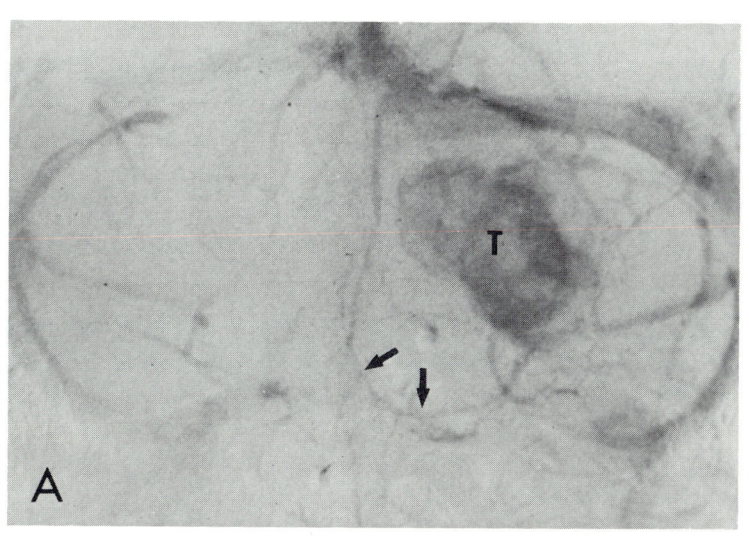
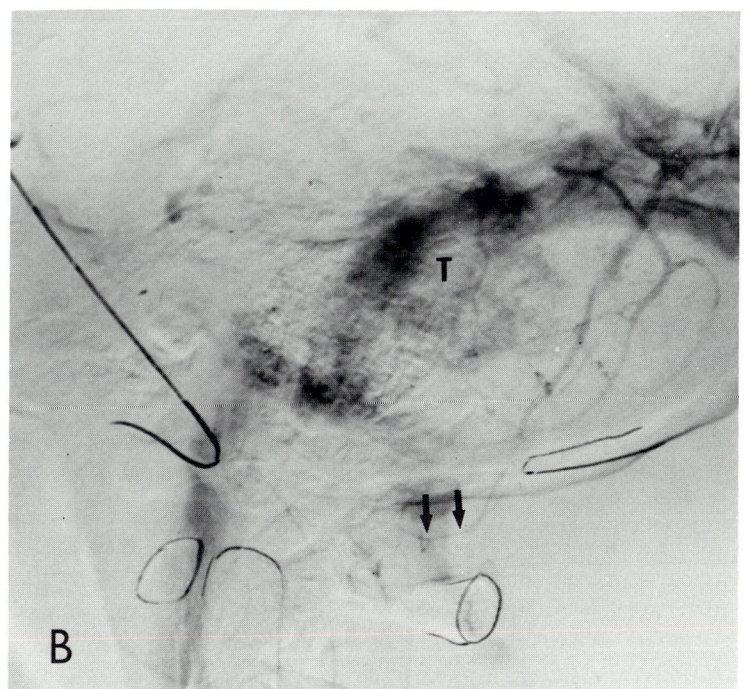

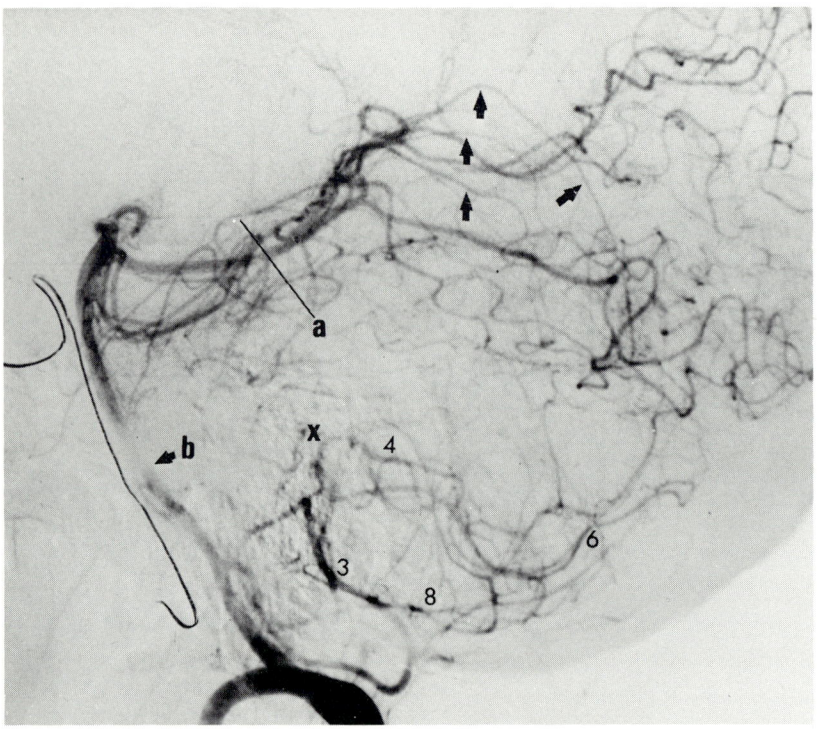

Fig. 8-13. Left cerebellar hemispheric metastasis from carcinoma of the colon. Left vertebral angiogram, arterial phase, lateral projection: same case as in Figs. 8-14, 8-15. The basilar artery (b) is displaced against the clivus. The posterior medullary segment (3) of PICA and the choroidal point (x) are displaced anteriorly. There is stretching of the supratonsillar (4) and inferior vermian (6) segments. A large tonsillohemispheric branch (8) of PICA is also stretched and inferiorly displaced. The ambient segment (a) of the superior cerebellar artery is displaced above the level of the equivalent segment of the posterior cerebral artery, and the superior vermian and hemispheric branches (arrows) of the superior cerebellar artery are stretched. These changes indicate expansion of the superior cerebellar hemisphere.

meningiomas, the hemispheric branches of the superior cerebellar artery are displaced inferiorly.[17] Separation of the superior vermian vein from the straight sinus also indicates an extracerebellar growth.[16] When the tumor originates from the tentorial edge, vessels within the ambient cistern are displaced in opposite directions. The posterior cerebral artery is then displaced superiorly and the superior cerebellar artery inferiorly.[21-23]

Rarely, the hemispheric branches of the superior cerebellar artery may

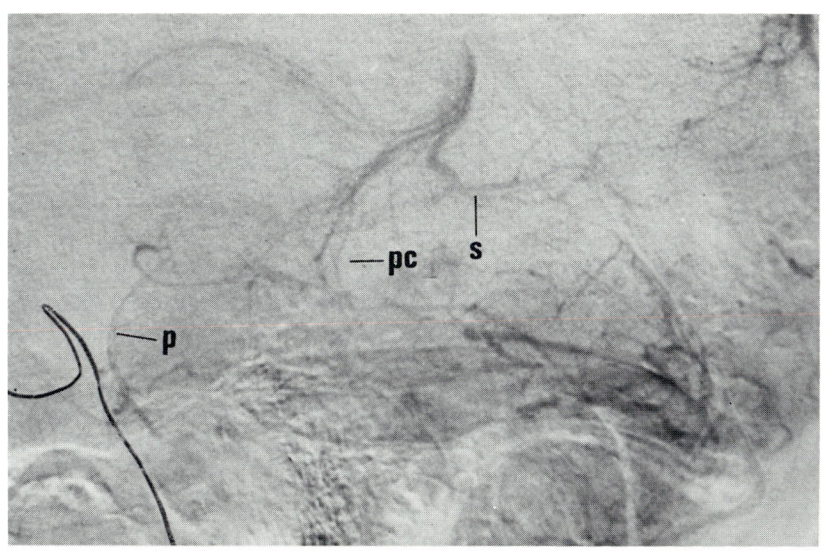

Fig. 8-14. Venous phase, lateral projection. The ponto-mesencephalic vein (p) is displaced anteriorly. The precentral cerebellar vein (pc) and the superior vermian vein (s) are also displaced anteriorly and superiorly indicating the presence of tumor in the cerebellar hemisphere.

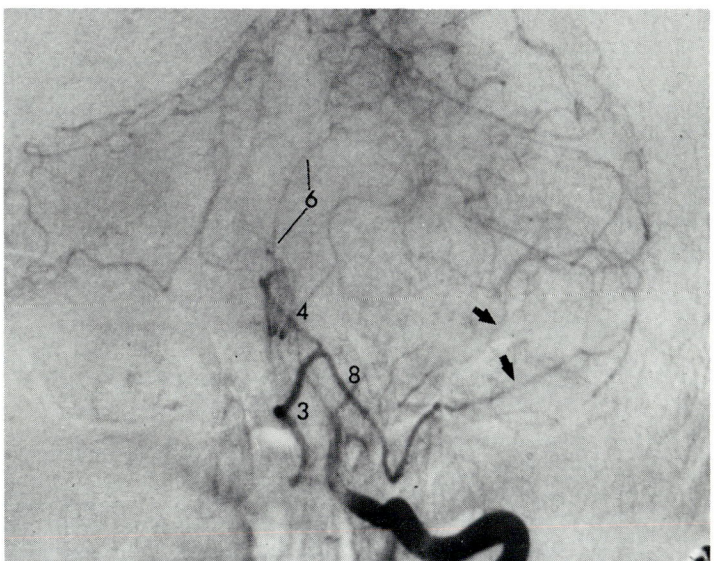

Fig. 8-15. Arterial phase, semiaxial projection. The posterior medullary segment (3) of PICA is displaced across the midline. The supratonsillar segment (4) is indicated. Note the stretching of the inferior vermian segment (6), the tonsillohemispheric branch (8), and the hemispheric tributaries (arrows).

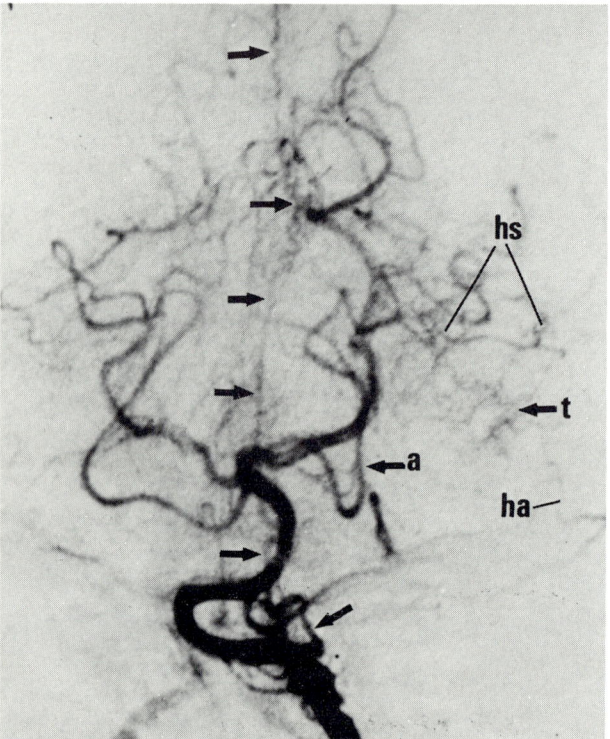

Fig. 8-16. Vascular superior cerebellar hemispheric metastasis from cerebellar hemispheric metastasis from carcinoma of the lung. Left vertebral angiogram, arterial phase, frontal projection: same case as Figs. 8-17 through 8-19. The ambient segment (a) of the left superior cerebellar artery is medially deviated. A vascular tumor stain (t) is seen supplied by hemispheric branches (hs) of the superior cerebellar artery and hemispheric branches (ha) of the anterior inferior cerebellar artery. Note the prominent, but normal, posterior meningeal branch of the vertebral artery (arrows).

apparently be occluded due to the tumor burrowing into the cerebellar hemisphere and compressing the vessels (Fig. 8-23A).

Primary tumors of the tentorium, such as meningiomas, frequently derive a blood supply from the tentorial artery (Fig. 8-26A,B).[24] The enlargement of the tentorial artery was initially thought to be specific for tentorial meningiomas, but subsequently many authors described enlargement of the tentorial artery in lesions other than meningiomas.[22,25-31] The enlargement in these

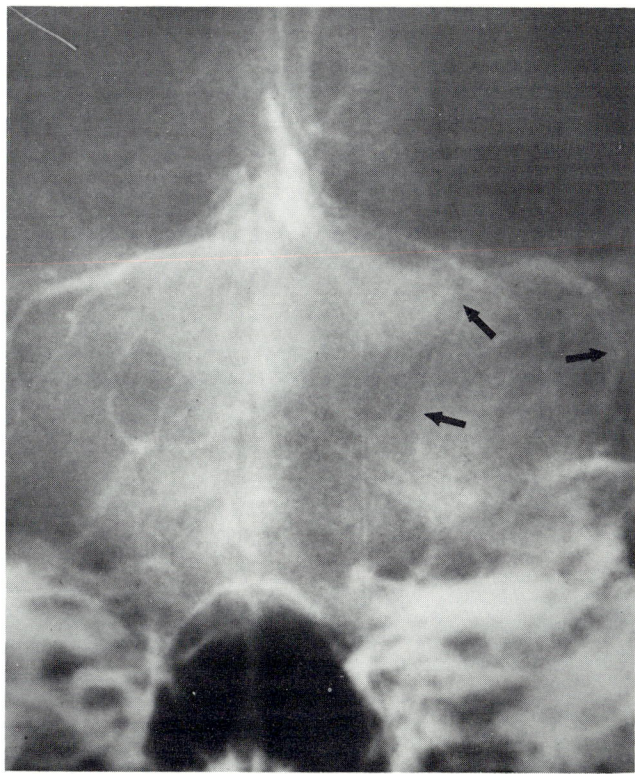

Fig. 8-17. Venous phase, frontal projection (non-subtracted film). Superior hemispheric veins (arrows) are stretched around the tumor.

cases is due to invasion of the tentorium from tumors of the adjacent brain and has been seen with gliomas, metastatic tumors, ependymomas, hemangioblastomas, and trigeminal neurinomas.

Frequently, it is necessary to perform selective internal carotid angiography to define the tentorial artery because, on common carotid angiography, the posterior branch of the middle meningeal artery can overlap the course of the tentorial artery.

When a meningioma originates from the posterior edge of the tentorium, it can simulate an intra-axial midbrain tumor with widening of the posterior cerebral arteries (Fig. 8-27A). Anterior displacement of the choroidal vessels and basal vein of Rosenthal, however, should suggest the correct diagnosis

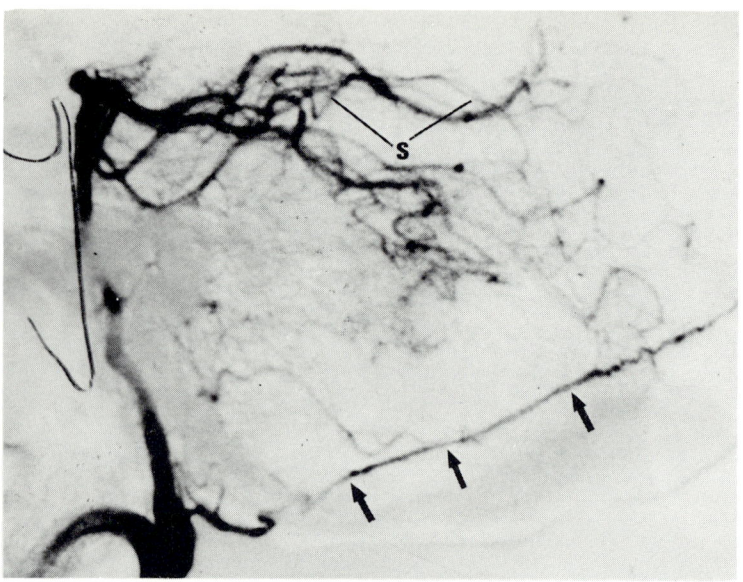

Fig. 8-18. Arterial phase, lateral projection. The superior vermian branch (s) of the superior cerebellar artery is displaced superiorly. Note the prominent, but normal, posterior meningeal branch of the vertebral artery (arrows).

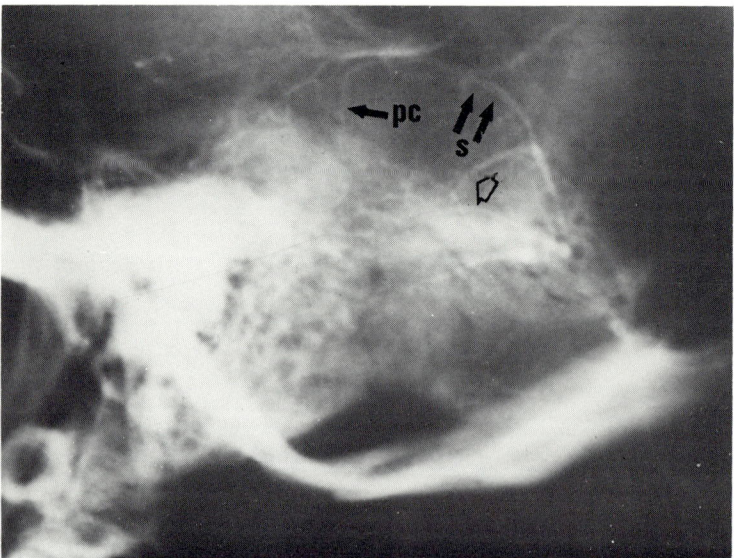

Fig. 8-19. Venous phase, lateral projection (non-subtracted film). The precentral cerebellar vein (pc) is displaced anteriorly, the superior vermian vein (s) superiorly, and there is stretching of a superior hemispheric vein (open arrow).

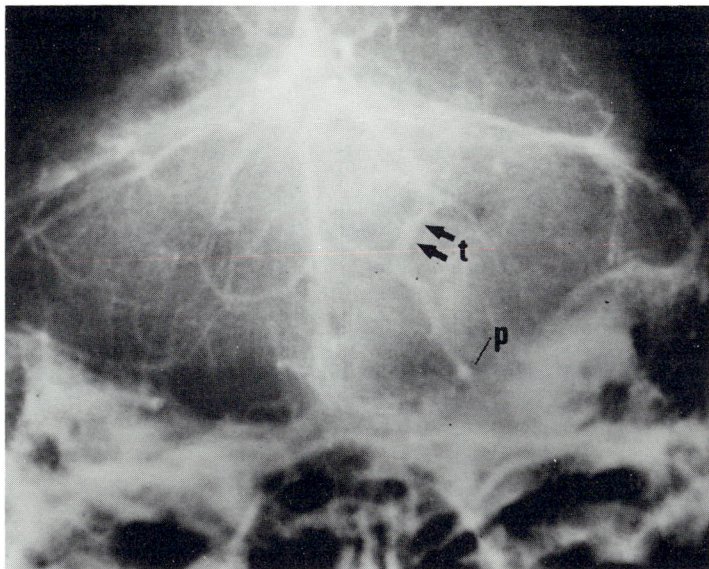

Fig. 8-20. Left cerebellar hemispheric metastasis from carcinoma of the lung. Left vertebral angiogram, venous phase, frontal projection (non-subtracted film). The brachial vein (t) is compressed by the tumor. Note the communication through the lateral anastomotic mesencephalic vein to the petrosal vein (p).

(Figs. 8-27B, 8-28). Arachnoid cysts, pineal tumors, and aneurysms of the great vein of Galen can cause similar displacements.[32]

When tumors originate outside the cerebellar hemisphere but invade the cerebellar hemisphere secondarily, they generally derive their blood supply from meningeal branches (Figs. 8-24A,B, 8-25). Dilatation of the occipital artery in meningiomas (Fig. 8-24A) suggests their extra-axial origin.[23,33-35]

Similarly, the posterior meningeal branch of the vertebral artery may be enlarged with meningiomas (Fig. 8-29). Since any tumor adjacent to the dura can cause enlargement of the posterior meningeal branch, the enlargement is not specific for meningiomas. The enlargement has also been described in cerebellar hemangioblastomas.[36-38]

Obstruction of the sinuses by tumor invasion is also suggestive of the extra-axial location of a tumor (Fig. 8-30). In addition to meningiomas, obstruction of the sinuses has been described in a case of rhabdomyosarcoma originating from the petrous bone.[39] Furthermore, the sinuses may be obstructed in cases of glomus jugulare tumors and in cases of sinus thrombosis secondary to adjacent mastoid infection. In view of the normal predilection to

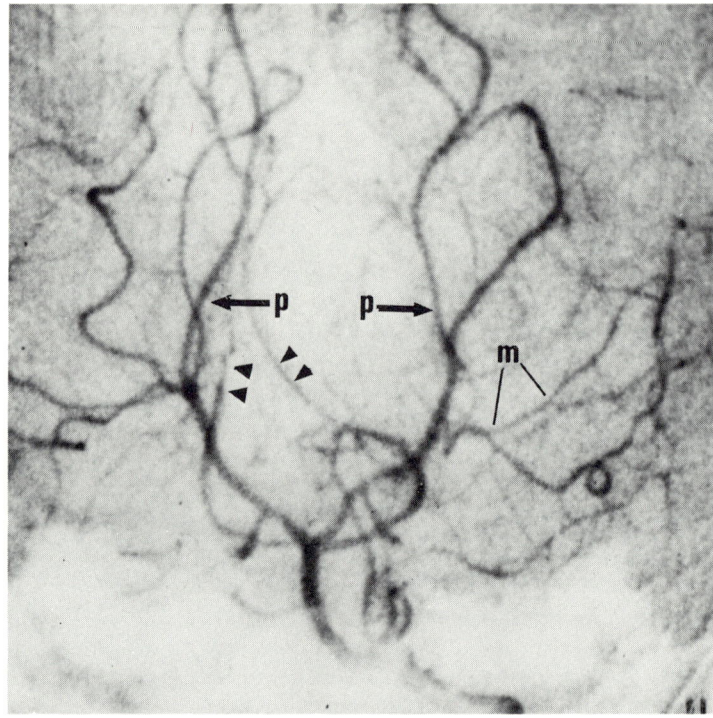

Fig. 8-21. Left superior hemispheric astrocytoma. Left vertebral angiogram, arterial phase, frontal projection: same case as in Fig. 8-22. The quadrigeminal segments of the posterior cerebral arteries (p) are markedly separated by upward herniation of the underlying tumor. The quadrigeminal segments of both superior cerebellar arteries (arrowheads) are deviated to the right side. The marginal branch (m) of the left superior cerebellar artery is stretched and displaced downward.

unequal transverse sinus size and opacification in carotid and vertebral angiography, nonfilling of a sinus must be critically evaluated before being considered pathological.

REFERENCES

1. Huang YP, Wolf BS: Angiographic features of fourth ventricle tumors with special reference to the posterior inferior cerebellar artery. Am J Roentgenol 107:543, 1969
2. Greitz T, Sjögren SE: The posterior inferior cerebellar artery. Acta Radiol [Diagn] (Stockh) 1:284, 1963

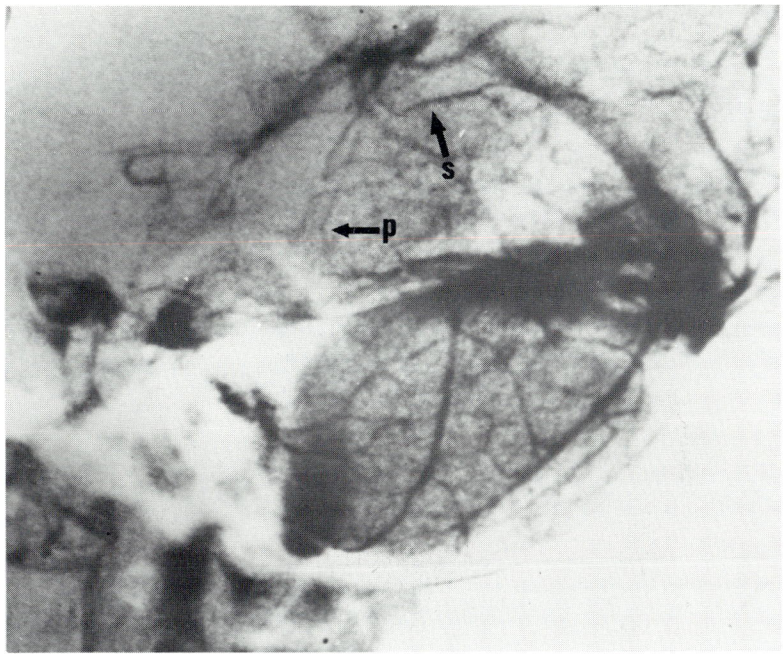

Fig. 8-22. Venous phase, lateral projection. The precentral cerebellar vein (p) is displaced anteriorly, while the superior vermian vein (s) is displaced superiorly.

3. Wolf BS, Newman CM, Khilnani MT: The posterior inferior cerebellar artery on vertebral angiography. Am J Roentgenol 87:322, 1962
4. Dufour M, Legré J: Aspects Neuro-radiologiques du diagnostic des tumeurs de la fosse postérieure. Ann Radiol (Paris) 12:473, 1969
5. Wilner HI, Navarro E, Bradley A, Eisenbrey B, Gracias V: The inferior vermian veins as a useful adjunct in the differentiation of brain stem tumors from midline cerebellar masses. Am J Roentgenol 108:605, 1973
6. Hauge T: Catheter vertebral angiography. Acta Radiol (Suppl) (Stockh) 109, 1954
7. Economos D, Prosalentis A: L'artère Cerebelleuse superieure dans les tumeurs de la Fosse Posterieure. Acta Radiol [Diagn] (Stockh) 1:267, 1963
8. Takahashi M, Wilson G, Hanafee W: Catheter vertebral angiography: a review of 300 examinations. J Neurosurg 30:722, 1969
9. Bull J, Kozlowski P: The angiographic pattern of the petrosal veins in the normal and pathological. Neuroradiology 1:20, 1970
10. Takahashi M: Atlas of Vertebral Angiography. Tokyo, Igaku Shoin, Ltd, 1974
11. Takahashi M, Okudera T, Fukui M, Kitamura K: The choroidal and nodular branches of the posterior inferior cerebellar artery. Their value in the diagnosis of medulloblastomas. Radiology 103:347, 1972
12. Takahashi M, Okudera T, Tanaka M, Kitamura K, Yonemasu Y: Angiographic diagnosis of

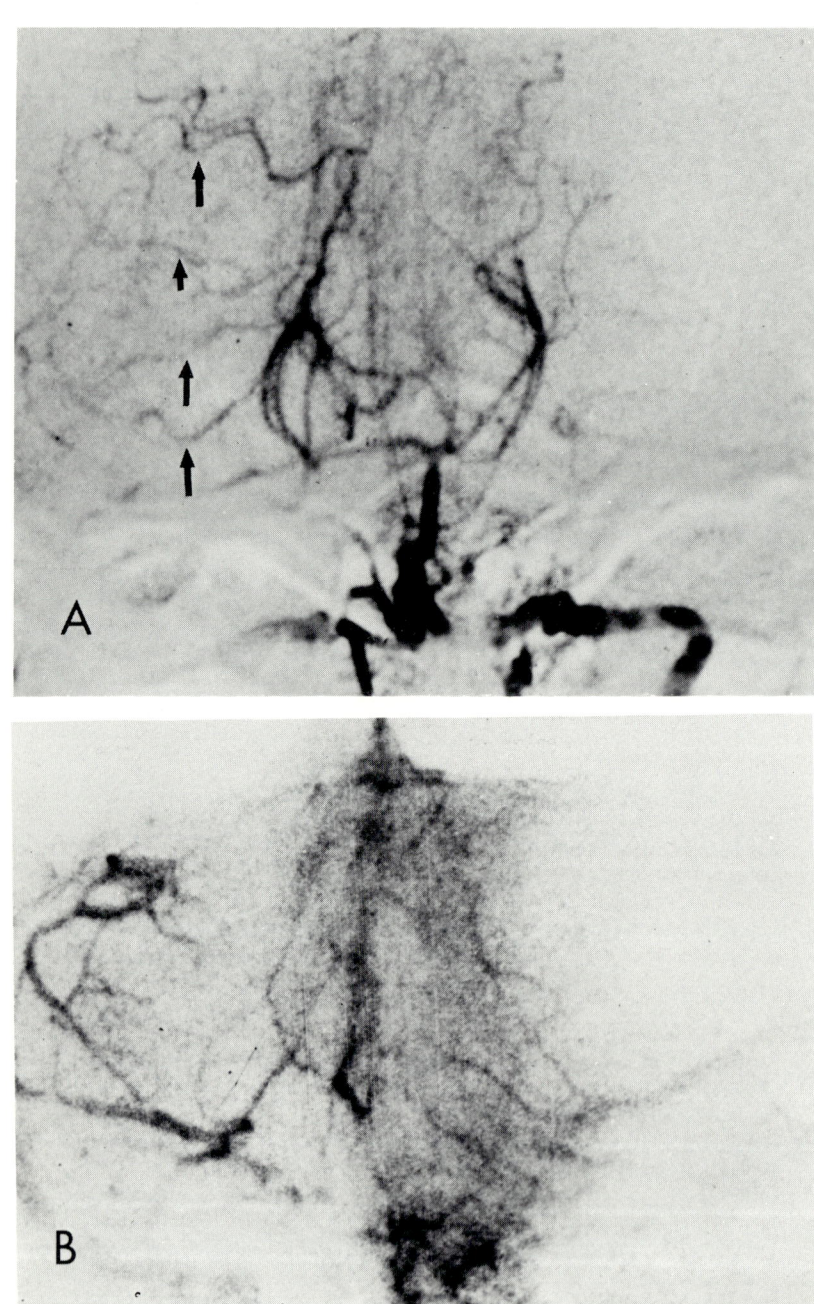

cerebellar medulloblastomas. Evaluation of pre- and postoperative vertebral angiographies. Am J Roentgenol 118:622, 1973
13. Russel DS, Rubinstein LJ: Pathology of Tumours of the Nervous System (ed 2). London, Arnold, 1963
14. Margolis MT, Newton TH: Borderlands of the normal and abnormal posterior inferior cerebellar artery. Acta Radiol [Diagn] (Stockh) 13:163, 1972
15. Margolis MT, Newton TH: An angiographic sign of cerebellar tonsillar herniation. Neuroradiology 2:3, 1971
16. Galligioni F, Bernardi R, Pellone M, Iraci G: The veins of the posterior cranial fossa: an angiographic study under pathologic conditions. Am J Roentgenol 110:39, 1970
17. Mani RL, Newton TH: The superior cerebellar artery: arteriographic changes in the diagnosis of posterior fossa lesions. Radiology 92:128, 1969
18. Löfgren FO: Vertebral angiography in the diagnosis of hydrocephalus and differentiation between stenosis of the aqueduct and cerebellar tumour. Acta Radiol 46:186, 1956
19. Huang YP, Wolf BS: The veins of the posterior fossa—superior or galenic draining group. Am J Roentgenol 95:808, 1965
20. Plaut HF: Vertebral and Carotid Angiograms in Tentorial Herniations; Including Roentgen Anatomy of the Tentorial Incisura. Springfield, Charles C Thomas, 1961
21. Greitz T: Tumours of the quadrigeminal plate and adjacent structures. Acta Radiol [Diagn] (Stockh) 12:513, 1972
22. Schechter MM, Zingesser LH, Rosenbaum A: Tentorial meningiomas. Am J Roentgenol 104:123, 1968
23. Pribram, HFW: The differentiation of extrinsic from intrinsic intracranial tumors with particular reference to posterior fossa tumors. Am J Roentgenol 98:542, 1966
24. Bernasconi V, Cassinari V: Un segno carotiografico tipico di meningioma del tentorio. Chirurgia 11:586, 1956, cited by Frugoni et al, Neurochir 2:142, 1960
25. Wallace S, Goldberg HI, Leeds NE, Mishkin MM: The cavernous branches of the internal carotid artery. Am J Roentgenol 101:34, 1967
26. Stattin S: Meningeal vessels of the internal carotid artery and their angiographic significance. Acta Radiol [Diagn] (Stockh) 55:329, 1961
27. Cortes O, Chase NE, Leeds N: Visualization of tentorial branches of the internal carotid artery in intracranial lesions other than meningiomas. Radiology 182:1024, 1964
28. Wirtala AO, Loop JW: Association of an enlarged tentorial artery with cerebellar hemangioblastoma. A case report. Radiology 96:67, 1970
29. El Gammal T, Roebuck EJ, du Boulay GH, Hoare RD: Further causes of hypertrophied tentorial arteries. Br J Radiol 40: 350, 1967
30. Kramer R, Newton TH: Tentorial branches of the internal carotid artery. Am J Roentgenol 95:826, 1965
31. Skultety FJ, Sorrell MF, Burklund CW: Hemangioblastoma of the cerebellum associated with erythrocytosis and an unusual blood supply. Case report. J Neurosurg 32:700, 1970

Fig. 8-23 A,B. Left tentorial meningioma burrowing into the cerebellar hemisphere. Left vertebral angiogram, arterial and venous phases, lateral projections: same case as Figs. 8-24A,B, 8-25. On the right side, the hemispheric and marginal branches (arrows) of the superior cerebellar artery are present, but they are obliterated on the left side. Similarly in the venous phase, hemispheric veins are present on the right, but absent on the left.

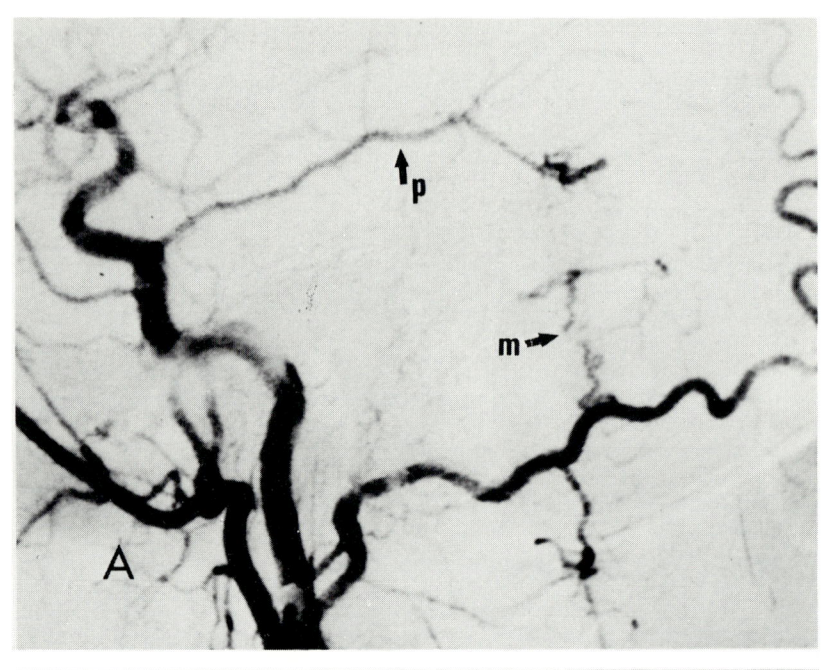
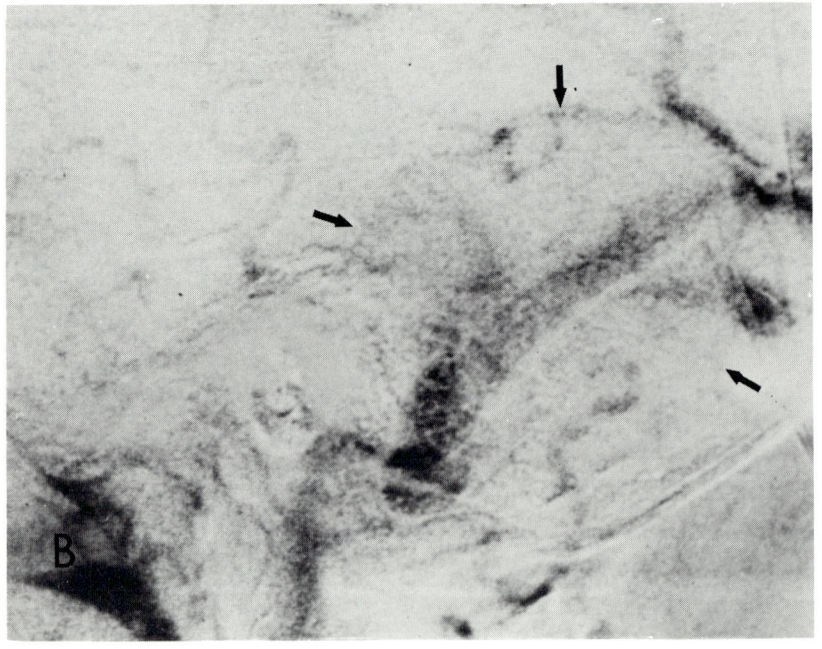

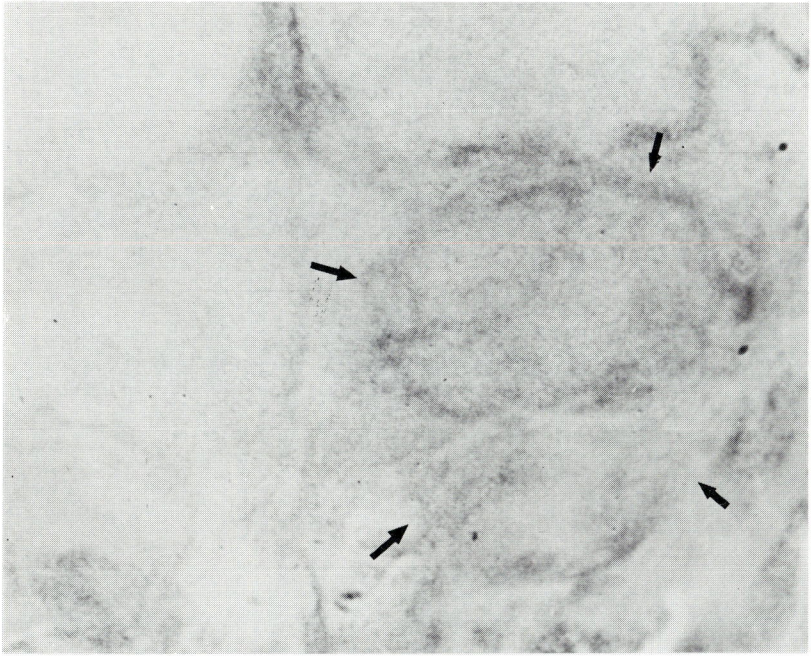

Fig. 8-25. Carotid angiogram, venous phase, frontal projection. The vascular stain of the meningioma (arrows) is seen which corresponds to the non-opacified area seen on the vertebral angiogram.

32. Newton TH, Margolis MT: Pathology involving the superior cerebellar artery, in Newton TH, Potts DG (eds): Radiology of the Skull and Brain, vol 2, book 2. St. Louis, Mosby, 1974 p 1831
33. Ruggiero G, Calabro A, Metzger J, Simon J: Arteriography of the external carotid artery. Acta Radiol [Diagn] (Stockh) 1:395, 1963
34. Nyström SHM, Nieminen JA: Angiographic findings in infratentorial fibromatous meningiomas. Ann Chir Gynaecol Fenn, 57:583, 1968
35. Salamon GM, Combalbert A, Raybaud C, Gonzalez J: An angiographic study of meningiomas of the posterior fossa. J Neurosurg 35:731, 1971

Fig. 8-24A,B. Left common carotid angiogram, arterial and venous phases, lateral projections. The posterior branch (p) of the middle meningeal artery is hypertrophied. Enlarged meningeal branches (m) are also seen originating from the occipital artery. In the venous phase, a faint stain (arrows) indicative of the meningioma can be seen.

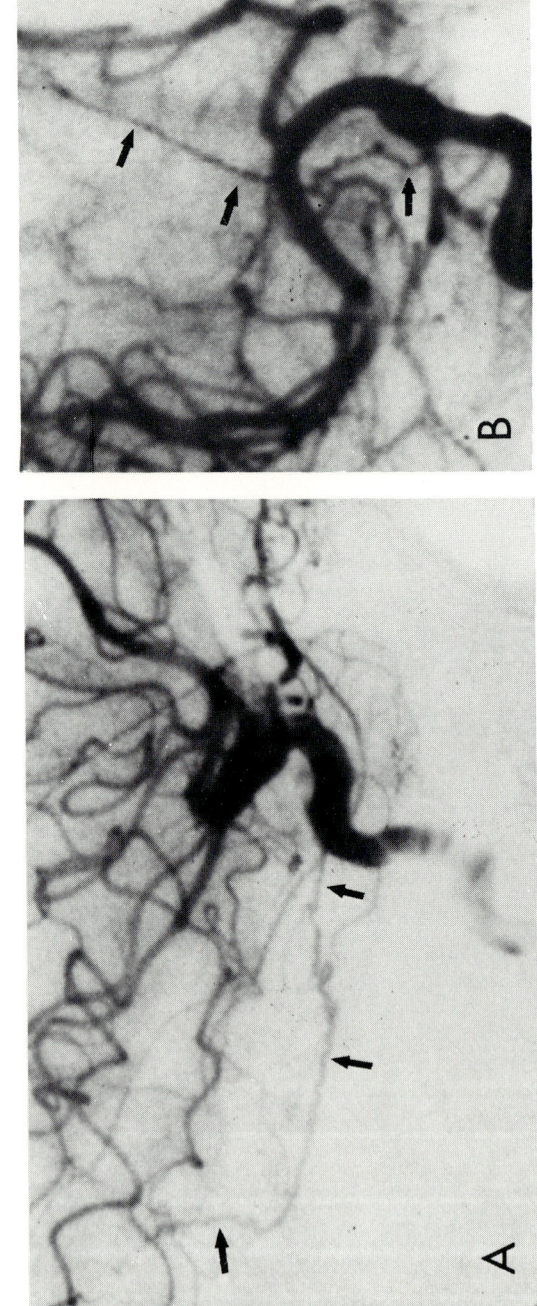

Fig. 8-26A,B. Tentorial meningioma originating from the posterior lip of the tentorium. Right internal carotid angiogram, arterial phase, lateral and frontal projections; same case as Figs. 8-27A,B, 8-28. The tentorial artery (arrows) is enlarged and supplies the tentorial meningioma.

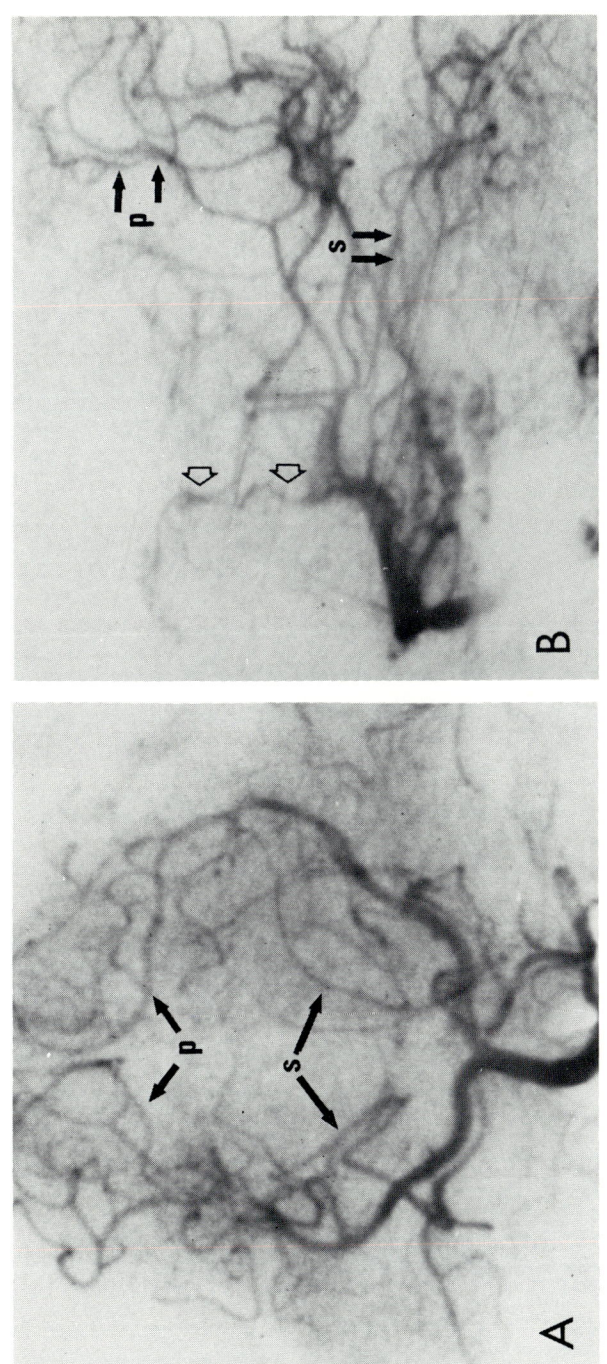

Fig. 8-27A,B. Left vertebral angiogram, arterial phase, frontal and lateral projections. The quadrigeminal segments of the superior cerebellar arteries (s) are depressed downward and markedly separated. The quadrigeminal segments of the posterior cerebral arteries (p) are also separated and are displaced backward. The posterior choroidal arteries (open arrows) are displaced anteriorly by the tumor.

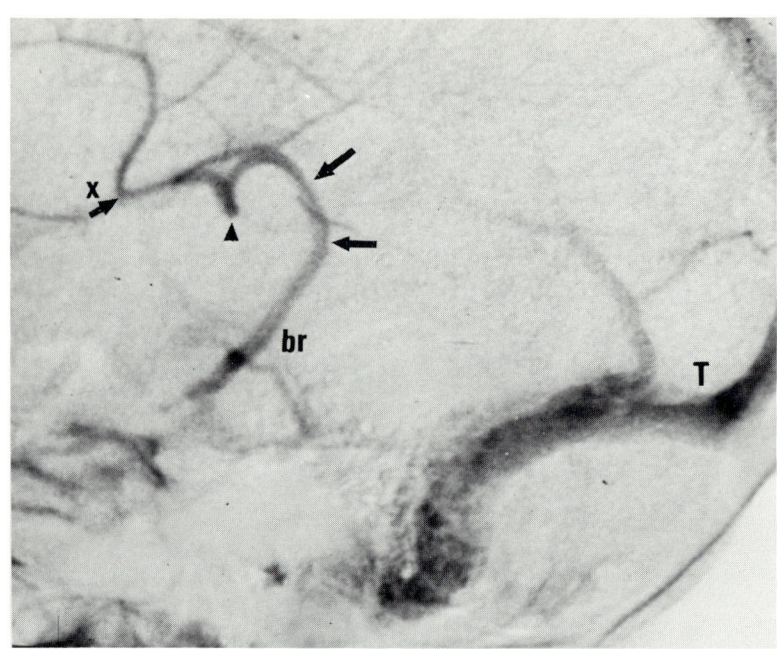

Fig. 8-28. Left carotid angiogram, venous phase, lateral projection. The basal vein of Rosenthal (br) at its junction with the internal cerebral vein (arrows) is markedly displaced forward by the tumor. As a result, the internal cerebral vein is kinked (arrowhead). The torcula (T) and the venous angle (x) are indicated.

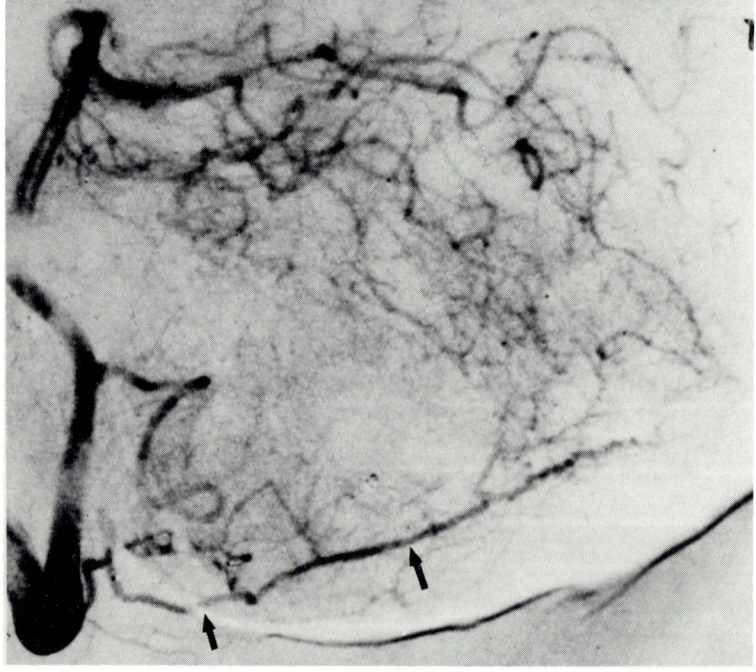

Vermian and Hemispheric Tumors

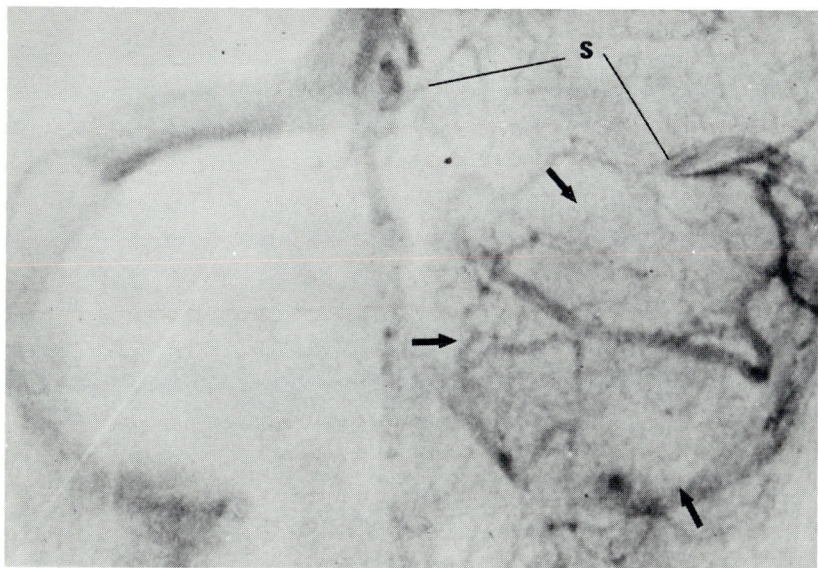

Fig. 8-30. Venous phase, frontal projection. The sigmoid sinus (s) is occluded by the tumor. The sinus was not seen on either carotid angiogram. Note the tumor stain (arrows).

36. Newton TH: The anterior and posterior meningeal branches of the vertebral artery. Radiology 91:271, 1968
37. Hawkins TD, Melcher DH: A meningeal artery in the falx cerebelli. Clin Radiol 17:377, 1966
38. Wolpert SM: The neuroradiology of hemangioblastomas of the cerebellum. Am J Roentgenol 110:56, 1970
39. Harwood-Nash DC: The radiology of rhabdomyosarcomas of the middle ear with intracranial extension in children. Clin Radiol 22:321, 1971

Fig. 8-29. Tentorial meningioma originating from attachment of the tentorium to the occipital squamosa. Left vertebral angiogram, arterial phase, lateral projection: same case as Fig. 8-30. The posterior meningeal branch (arrows) of the vertebral artery is enlarged. Often, this is difficult to appreciate since the artery normally may be surprisingly prominent (see Fig. 8-18).

9
Differential Diagnosis of Posterior Fossa Tumors

Certain characteristics of the radiology of a tumor in the posterior fossa as demonstrated by vertebral angiography allow the physician, in most instances, to arrive at the correct pathological diagnosis. The diagnosis is derived from a combined consideration of the age of the patient, the appearances of the skull X-ray, the location of the tumor, and finally the angioarchitecture of the tumor.

Standard neuroradiological texts have fully covered the plain skull X-ray appearances of posterior fossa tumors.[1,2] Bone erosion, bone thinning, hyperostosis, calcification, and soft tissue densities should always be carefully looked for as they can provide valuable clues as to the site and nature of the underlying tumor. Consideration of the patient's age and the location of the tumor also allow the nature of the tumor to be predicted with a fair degree of certainty (see Chapter 3).

This chapter reviews the angioarchitecture of the tumors and to what degree these features are pathologically significant.

ACOUSTIC NEURINOMAS

Tumor stains may be seen with acoustic neurinomas (see Figs. 5-13, 5-15).[3,4] The stains are presumably due to opacification of the tumor by branches of the internal auditory and anterior inferior cerebellar arteries, although on occasion, such stains have only been seen after opacification of the external carotid artery.[5] The tumor stain of an acoustic neurinoma has been described as faint and patchy; in contrast, that of a meningioma is usually homogeneous and is present from the arterial through to the venous phase of the angiogram.[6] Tortuous, irregular tumor vessels with intermixed areas of increased and decreased vascularity simulating malignant gliomas were seen in benign neurinomas of the head and neck, including acoustic neurinomas, by Moscow and Newton.[7] On occasions, the vascular stains are best seen by adopting an oblique frontal projection with the patient's head turned away from the side of injection.[8] Subtraction techniques are of major value in demonstrating the faint tumor stain of an acoustic neurinoma, since many apparently avascular acoustic neurinomas are shown to be faintly vascular on the subtraction films. Acoustic neurinomas have been described in which the blood supply is exclusively from the dorsal clival branch of the internal carotid artery and the middle meningeal artery.[9] Accordingly, the evaluation of a patient with a suspected acoustic neurinoma should include angiography of the vertebral artery, the internal carotid artery, and the external carotid artery.

When an acoustic neurinoma is particularly vascular, the anterior inferior cerebellar artery may be enlarged, and arteriovenous shunting may occur (see Figs. 5-14, 5-15). Early draining veins are often present within the capsule of the tumor and can accurately outline its size.[6]

MENINGIOMAS

Whereas supratentorial meningiomas frequently are diagnosed by the presence of a homogeneous blush present from the later arterial through to the venous phase of an angiogram, according to some authors, this feature is not as common in infratentorial meningiomas. In one series of eight infratentorial fibromatous meningiomas investigated by both carotid and vertebral angiography, no vascular stains were encountered.[10] Schechter and co-workers as well as Ruggiero and co-workers, however, described vascular stains indistinguishable from those seen in supratentorial meningiomas in their cases of tentorial meningiomas.[11,12] Hoffman and associates described a vascular stain in a case of fourth ventricle meningioma.[13] A similar case with enlargement of the choroidal branches of PICA was described by Rodriguez-Carbajal and Palacios.[14]

"Pathological vessels" in meningiomas were described by Radner and Hauge.[15,16]

The major blood supply to meningiomas of the posterior fossa is from the external carotid artery. In a series of seventeen posterior fossa meningiomas of all pathological types, Salamon and associates described enlarged meningeal vessels derived from the external carotid artery as well as tumor stains as constant radiological features (see Figs. 5-5A,B, 8-24A,B, 8-25, 8-30).[17] In the eight cases of cerebellar convexity meningiomas described by Kendall and

Shah, the blood supply was from the external carotid artery in seven cases and from the meningeal branches of the vertebral artery in only one case.[18] On occasions, the major blood supply is from the meningohypophyseal branch of the internal carotid artery (see Figs. 5-6A,B, 5-7, 5-20, 8-26A,B).

Kendall and Shah also described upper bulging of the tentorium, diagnosed by bowing of the straight sinus, as a significant diagnostic sign in their cases of meningiomas.[18] This sign was not seen with intrinsic cerebellar hemispheric masses, but was seen, on occasions, with acoustic neurinomas.

FIFTH NERVE NEURINOMAS

Abnormal tumor vessels and spotty accumulation of contrast material have been described in fifth nerve neurinomas.[16,19] Usually, however, these tumors are avascular.

HEMANGIOBLASTOMAS

The value of angiography in the diagnosis of cerebellar hemangioblastomas has been stressed by many authors.[1,15,16,20-23] The angiographic appearances can vary, but the most common appearance is that of a dense nodular tumor stain often with irregular central translucencies (see Fig. 8-12A,B). On occasion, the nodule may be homogeneous throughout. A second type of lesion seen less frequently than the first type is that of a tangle of vessels resembling an arteriovenous malformation (see Figs. 8-1A,B, 8-2). Again, this latter type of lesion may have a translucent center or be homogeneous throughout. The presence of an adjacent avascular cyst causing considerable vessel displacement is a very useful adjunctive radiological sign. This may occur with either type. Enlarged feeding arteries and draining veins can occur in both types. The differential diagnosis from an arteriovenous malformation may then be extremely difficult.[24] On occasion, tentorial arteries can provide a major blood supply to the tumor.[25-27]

GLOMUS JUGULARE TUMORS

On angiography, these tumors usually demonstrate a blush in the region of the jugular fossa or in the middle ear. According to Hawkins, the angiographic pattern consists of an irregular network of small vessels with pooling of contrast agent in vascular lakes.[28] An arteriovenous shunt may also be seen. The correct diagnosis can be determined from the typical bone changes and the blood supply from the ascending pharyngeal artery.[29] (See Chapter 5.)

MISCELLANEOUS TUMORS

The remaining infratentorial tumors are generally avascular, and their presence can only be determined by vascular displacements. A case of a vascular medulloblastoma, however, with arteriovenous shunts and early venous filling has been reported.[24] Pathological arterial vessels (hypertrophied arteries of irregular size and shape) generally are not seen in infratentorial tumors, though pathological arterial branches have been described in medulloblastomas.[30] These branches may be identical to the nodular vessels derived from the supratonsillar segment of PICA described by Takahashi and co-workers in cases of medulloblastomas (see Fig. 7-6A).[31] Pathological tumor stains have also been described in astrocytomas.[32]

Metastatic tumors to the cerebellum that are vascular usually originate in the kidney or thyroid gland. We have also seen cases of vascular metastatic tumors from anaplastic carcinomas of the lung (see Figs. 8-16, 8-17). Rarely, an ependymoma may present as a vascular tumor.

Glioblastomas multiforme are rare tumors in the posterior fossa, but when present may have enlarged feeding arteries and draining veins.[32]

REFERENCES

1. Taveras JM, Wood EH: Diagnostic Neuroradiology. Baltimore, Williams & Wilkins, 1964
2. Newton TH, Potts DG (eds): Radiology of the Skull and Brain, vol 1, books 1 and 2. St. Louis, Mosby, 1971
3. Takahashi M, Okudera T, Tomanaga M, Kitamura K: Angiographic diagnosis of acoustic neurinomas: analysis of 30 lesions. Neuroradiology 2:191, 1971
4. Des Plantes ZBG: X-Ray examination in cerebellopontine angle tumours. Psychiatria Neurol Neurochir 71:133, 1968
5. Levine HL, Ferris EJ, Spatz EL: External carotid blood supply to acoustic neurinomas. Report of two cases. J Neurosurg 38:516, 1973
6. Symon L, Kendall B: The use of vertebral angiography in the differential diagnosis of cerebello-pontine angle lesions, in Schürmann K, Brock M, Reulen H-J, Voth D (eds): Advances in Neurosurgery, vol 1. Berlin, Springer-Verlag, 1973
7. Moscow NP, Newton TH: Angiographic features of hypervascular neurinomas of the head and neck. Radiology 114:635, 1975
8. Huang YP, Wolf BS, Anten SP, et al: Angiographic features of cerebellopontine angle tumors. Ninth Annual Meeting of American Society of Neuroradiology. San Francisco, 1971
9. Théron J, Lasjaunias P: Participation of the external and internal carotid arteries in the vascular supply of cerebellopontine angle tumours. Thirteenth Annual Meeting of American Society of Neuroradiology, Vancouver, 1975
10. Nyström SHM, Nieminen JA: Angiographic findings in infratentorial fibromatous meningiomas. Ann Chir Gynaecol Fenn 57:583, 1968
11. Schechter MM, Zingesser LH, Rosenbaum A: Tentorial Meningiomas. Am J Roentgenol 104:123, 1968

12. Ruggiero G, Calabro A, Metzger J, Simon J: Arteriography of the external carotid artery. Acta Radiol [Diagn] (Stockh) 1:395, 1963
13. Hoffman JC, Bufkin WJ, Richardson HD: Primary intraventricular meningiomas of the fourth ventricle. Am J Roentgenol 115:100, 1972
14. Rodriguez-Carbajal J, Palacios E: Intraventricular meningiomas of the fourth ventricle. Am J Roentgenol 120:27, 1974
15. Radner S: Vertebral angiography by catheterization. A new method employed in 221 cases. Acta Radiol (Suppl) (Stockh) 87, 1951
16. Hauge T: Catheter vertebral angiography. Acta Radiol (Suppl) (Stockh) 109, 1954
17. Salamon GM, Combalbert A, Raybaud C, Gonzalez J: An angiographic study of meningiomas of the posterior fossa. J Neurosurg 35:731, 1971
18. Kendall B, Shah S: Investigation of meningiomas of cerebellar convexities. Neuroradiology 4:162, 1972
19. Westberg G: Angiographic changes in neurinoma of the trigeminal nerve. Acta Radiol [Diagn] (Stockh) 1:513, 1963
20. Krayenbühl HA, Yaşargil MG: Cerebral Angiography (ed 2). Philadelphia, Lippincott, 1968
21. Sjögren SE: Percutaneous vertebral angiography: review of 250 cases. Acta Radiol 40:113, 1953
22. Ollson O: Vertebral angiography in cerebellar haemangioma. Acta Radiol 40:9, 1953
23. Wolpert SM: The neuroradiology of hemangioblastomas of the cerebellum. Am J Roentgenol 110:56, 1970
24. Anacker H, Strehele H: Die Angiographie der A. vertebralis durch selektive Katheterisierung und ihre Ergebnisse. Fortschr Geb Roentgenstr Nuklearmed 107:169, 1967
25. Wirtala AO, Loop JW: Association of an enlarged tentorial artery with cerebellar hemangioblastoma. A case report. Radiology 96:67, 1970
26. El Gammal T, Roebuck EJ, du Boulay GH, Hoare RD: Further causes of hypertrophied tentorial arteries. Br J Radiol 40:350, 1967
27. Skultety FM, Sorrell MF, Burklund CW: Hemangioblastomas of the cerebellum associated with erythrocytosis and an unusual blood supply. Case report. J Neurosurg 32:700, 1970
28. Hawkins TD: Glomus jugulare and carotid body tumours. Clin Radiol 12:199, 1961
29. Palacios E: Chemodectomas of the head and neck. Am J Roentgenol 110:129, 1970
30. La Torre E, Occhipinti E, Pollicita A: Retrograde brachial angiography in the diagnosis of infratentorial tumor in infancy and childhood. Eur Neurol 4:77, 1970
31. Takahashi M, Okudera T, Fukui M, Kitamura K: The choroidal and nodular branches of the posterior inferior cerebellar artery. Their value in the diagnosis of medulloblastomas. Radiology 103:347, 1972
32. Takahashi M: Atlas of Vertebral Angiography. Tokyo, Igaku Shoin, Ltd, 1974

Index

Acoustic neurinomas, 21, 26, 28, 91
  angiographic appearance, *106, 107*
  angiography of vertebral artery, and carotid artery, 177
    diagnostic accuracy, 104
  arteriovenous shunts, 101, *107*, 177
  basilar artery displacement, 104, *110, 111, 112*
  blood supply, 100, 177
  clinical aspects, 21
  differential diagnosis, 176–177
  early draining veins, 177
  pathology, 26
  tumor stains, *106, 107,* 176
  vascular displacement, 100, 101, *105, 108*
AICA. *See* Anterior inferior cerebellar artery
Anastomosis
  congenital, between carotid and basilar arteries, 70
  occipitovertebral, 48
Angiographic anatomy
  basilar artery, 52–70
    anterior inferior cerebellar artery, 32–33, 54–61
    branches, 52–54
    labyrinthine artery (internal auditory artery), 61–62
    pontine arteries, 61
    posterior cerebral arteries, 64–69
      anterior temporal artery, 65
      cortical branches, 65
      parieto-occipital and calcarine arteries, 66–67
      penetrating branches, 67
      posterior choroidal arteries, 68–69
      posterior pericallosal artery, 67
      posterior temporal artery, 65
      quadrigeminal and geniculate body arteries, 67
      thalamoperforating arteries, 67
    superior cerebellar arteries, 32–33, 62–64
      hemispheric arteries, 62
      marginal artery, 62
      superior vermian artery, 62–64
    variations, 69–70
  cervical epidural venous system, 75
  cervicovertebral veins, 73
  color plate diagrams, *33–34*
    fourth ventricle tumors (Plate V), *34*–35
    inferior vermian and hemispheric tumors (Plate VI), *34*–35
    normal inferior cerebellar anatomy (Plate I), *32–33*
    normal superior cerebellar anatomy (Plate II), *32–33*
    pontine and mesencephalic tumors (Plate IV), *34*–35
    prepontine and cerebellopontine angle tumors (Plate III), *32–33*
    superior vermian and hemispheric tumors, (Plate VII), *34*–35
  inferior vermian vein, *55,* 84, 122
    variations, 87
  jugular vein, 73
  meningeal arteries, 71–73
    anterior branch, 71

Angiographic anatomy *(continued)*
 anterosuperior group, 71–72
 branches of ascending pharyngeal artery, 38, 73, *95, 98*
 dorsal, 72, *99*
 inferior group, 71
 inferior hypophyseal artery, 72
 lateral group, 72
 meningeal branch of occipital artery, 72
 posterior branch, 71
 posterior branch of middle meningeal artery, 72
 recurrent branches of middle meningeal artery, 72
 tentorial artery, 72
 normal anatomy, 31–90
 ponto-mesencephalic veins, 18, 76, 85–86, *96*
 variations, 85
 posterior fossa veins, 75–84
  anterior (petrosal) group, 75–76
  brachial veins, 76
  cerebellomedullary veins, 77
  inferior vermian veins, 84
  petrosal vein, 77–79
  ponto-mesencephalic vein, 76
  posterior mesencephalic veins, 79
  posterior (tentorial) group, 83
  precentral cerebellar vein, 81–83
  superior and inferior hemispheric veins, 76
  superior (Galenic) group, 79
  superior vermian vein, 83
  vein of lateral recess of fourth ventricle, 76–77
 precentral cerebellar vein, 81–83
 variations, 86
 spinal cord veins, 75
 suboccipital venous plexus, 74–75
 supratentorial veins, 84–87
  basal vein of Rosenthal, 84
  choroid plexus and superior choroidal veins, 85
  internal cerebral vein, 85
  occipital veins, 85
  thalamic veins, 85
 vertebral artery, 31–52
  anterior spinal artery, 39
  cervical branches, 38
  intracranial branches, 38
  medullary arteries, 40
  meningeal arteries, 38
  muscular branches, 38
  posterior inferior cerebellar artery, 40–47
  posterior spinal artery, 40
  spinal branches, 38
  variations, 47–52
 vertebral vein, 73–74
Anesthesia for angiographic technique, 4
Aneurysms
 anterior inferior cerebellar artery, 91
 basilar artery, 91
 vertebral artery, 91
Angiography. *See also* Vertebral angiographic techniques
 angiotomography to define midline vessels, 18
 brachial, 2, 8
 explaining to patients, 4
 historical aspects, 1–3
 preoperative evaluation, 27–29
 sedation, 4–5
 subclavian, 8
 techniques, 4–19
 value of, 29
 vertebral. *See* Vertebral angiography
Angiotome, 18
Angiotomography, 18
 side-to-side rotation of head, 18
Anterior cerebral artery, 65*n*
Anterior communicating artery, 65*n*
Anterior condyloid foramen (hypoglossal canal), 48
Anterior inferior cerebellar artery (AICA), 26, 28, 54–61, *107*
 aneurysms, 91
 angiographic anatomy, 32–*33*, *49*, 54–59, *60*, 61
 variations, 48, 69–70
 Caldwell projection, *60, 61, 97*, 100, *103*
 cerebellopontine angle tumors, *60, 97*, 100, *102, 103, 111*
 course of, 28, *41*, 51
 fifth cranial nerve neurinomas, 101
 normal anatomy, 32
 pontine and mesencephalic tumors, *119, 121*
 radiographic studies, 28
 site of origin, *41, 60*
 tumor stains, 176
 undulant curves, 51
Anterior meningeal branch, *39*, 71, 97
 prepontine tumors, *94, 95*

Index

Anterior ponto-mesencephalic vein, 18
Anterior spinal artery, *37, 39, 51*
　normal anatomy, 51
　pontine and mesencephalic tumors, 118
Anterior temporal artery, *59,* 65, *66*
Aqueduct, 20, *64*
　Sahlstedt's point for, 46
Arachnoid cysts, 91, 165
　congenital, 106
Arnold-Chiari malformation, 151
Arteries. *See specific arteries*
Arteriovenous fistula, complicating vertebral angiography, 10
Arteriovenous shunts
　acoustic neurinomas, 101, *107*
　glomus jugulare tumors, 178
Ascending pharyngeal artery, 58, 73
　clival meningiomas, *98*
　glomus jugulare tumors and, 178
　meningeal branches, 73, 95, *98*
Astrocytomas, 115
　cerebellar, 129
　childhood tumors, 23, 25
　　involving brainstem, 25
　　involving cerebellar hemisphere, 23
　cystic, 23, 26, *152*
　left superior hemispheric, *166, 167*
　low-grade, 21, 23, 25
　pathology, 23, 25
　right inferior hemispheric, *153, 154, 155, 156, 167*
　tumor stains, 179
　vermian cystic, *152*
Ataxia, limb, 20–21, 22
Atherosclerosis
　subclavian angiography for, 8
　transaxillary catheterization of vertebral artery and, 2
Atherosclerotic vascular disease, selective catheterization avoided, 5
Atropine (atropine sulfate), 4
Audiological testing, 26
Auditory canal, internal, 55. *See also* Internal auditory canal
Axillary arteriotomies, complications, 10

Basal vein of Rosenthal, 84
　displaced by tumor, 163, 165, *173, 174*
　midbrain tumors, 120
　variations, 85–86
　vermian and hemispheric tumors, 163–165, *173, 174*
Basal venous plexus, *96*
Basilar artery
　acoustic neurinomas, 104, *110, 111, 112*
　aneurysms, 91
　angiographic anatomy, *37,* 52–70
　　anterior inferior cerebellar artery, 54–61
　　branches, 52–54
　　hypoplastic left vertebral artery, *57*
　　labyrinthine artery (internal auditory artery), 52, 61–62
　　pontine arteries, 52, 61, *117, 121*
　　posterior cerebral arteries, 52, 64
　　superior cerebellar arteries, 52, 62–64
　　supplied by right vertebral artery, *59*
　　from two vertebral arteries, 37, 52
　　variations, 69–70
　cerebellopontine angle tumors, 102–104
　fourth ventricle tumors, 129, *130,* 131, *135, 137, 138, 142, 143, 144*
　differential diagnosis of pontine from fourth ventricle tumors, 116
　meningiomas, 104, *110, 111, 112*
　pontine and mesencephalic tumors, 115–118, *117, 118*
　prepontine tumors, *92, 93, 94, 95, 96, 101*
　thrombosis, 11
　vermian and hemispheric tumors, 146, *148, 149, 150,* 153–154, *155, 156*
　visualization of, 11
Bleeding, complication of vertebral angiography, 9
Blindness, following angiography, 10–11
Blood vessels, angiotomography of, 18
Bone, erosion and thinning, 176
Brachial angiography, 2, 8
　with retrograde injection of contrast material, 2
Brachial artery, thrombosis, 9
Brachial plexus paralysis, 10
Brachial veins, 76
　superior vermian and hemispheric tumors, 156, *165*
　variations, 86
Brain scans, angiography and, 27
Brain tumors
　incidence, 22
Brainstem rotation, cerebellopontine angle tumors, 102
Brainstem tumors, 21

Brainstem tumors *(continued)*
  acoustic neurinomas, 26
  angiographic changes, 120–123
  anterior displacement, 153
  astrocytomas, 25, 115
  benign cysts or blood clots mimicking tumors, 29
  childhood tumors, 25
    astrocytoma, 25
  clinical aspects, 21
  compression in fourth ventricle tumors, 131
  eccentric low, 122
  gliomas, 29, 122
  high, 121–122
  intra-axial, 157
  low-grade glial tumors, 115
    posterior displacements, 120–122
  pathology, 25
  pontine glioma, *117, 118, 119, 120, 121*
  site of origin, 115
  surgical considerations, 26–29
British Journal of Radiology, 2
Bulbar movements, 21

Calcarine arteries, *44, 45, 58, 59,* 66–67
Calcification and differential diagnosis, 176
Caldwell projection, anterior inferior cerebellar artery, *60, 61, 97,* 100, *103*
Carcinomas of lungs
  metastatic tumors to cerebellum and, *162, 163, 165,* 179
  vermian and hemispheric tumors and, *162, 163, 164, 165*
Caroticotympanic artery, 105
  injections of contrast material, 1
Carotid artery, internal. *See* Internal carotid artery
Catheters and catherization
  for arterial catheterization, 5
  complications, 9–11
    manipulative, 10–11
  guide wires, 5–7, 10
  needle and catheter dimensions, 6
  nonthrombogenic arterial, 9
  soft Hanafee catheter, 10
  thromboembolism and size of catheters, 9
  vertebral artery, 1–2, 5, 31
Caudal loop, 40, 41, 49, 52, *92,* 102
  tonsillar herniation, *52,* 151
Central nervous system, astrocytoma tumors, 23, 25
Cerebellar arteries
  anterior inferior. *See* Anterior inferior cerebellar artery
  inferior. *See* Inferior cerebellar arteries
  posterior inferior. *See* Posterior inferior cerebellar articles
  superior. *See* Superior cerebellar arteries
Cerebellar convexity meningiomas, 92, 177–178
Cerebellar hemisphere tumors, 23
  astrocytoma, 23, 25, 129
    left superior, *166, 167*
    right inferior, *153, 154, 155, 156,* 157
  clinical and pathological aspects, 20
  hemangioblastomas, 26, *158,* 165
  pathology, 23
Cerebellar hemisphere, vermian and hemispheric tumors, 165
Cerebellar tonsil tumors, 147–151
  herniation of cerebellar tonsils, 151
  oligodendroglioma, *158*
Cerebellar vermis tumors
  clinical aspects, 20
  medulloblastoma, 23–24
  pathology, 23–24
Cerebellolabyrinthine arteries, 49
  stretching and displacement of, 100
Cerebellomedullary vein, 77
Cerebellopontine angle
  extra-axial masses, 91
  fourth ventricle tumors, 134, *141*
    differential diagnosis of pontine glioma from, 120
  meningiomas, 26
  surgical considerations, 27–28
Cerebellopontine angle tumors, 21, 25, 28, 91–114
  acoustic neurinomas, 91
  anatomy, 32–33
    brainstem rotation, 102
    cholesteatomas, 92
    clinical aspects, 21
    colored plate diagram, 32–33
    normal anatomy, 32–33
    surgical considerations, 27, 28
    vascular displacement, *97, 102, 111*
Cerebellum, precentral lobule, *64*
Cerebellum tumors, 20–21
  clinical aspects, 20–21
  hemangioblastomas, 25–26

Index

Cerebral arteries
 anterior, 65*n*
 posterior. *See* Posterior cerebral arteries
Cerebral spinal fluid (CSF)
 elevated protein, 25
 obstruction with hydrocephalus, 20–22
 surgical unblocking of passageways, 27
 ventriculography, 28
Cerebral veins
 angiographic anatomy, 73–78
  variations, 85–87
 internal, 85
Cervical cord, 38
 normal anatomy, *51*
Cervical epidural venous system, 75
Cervicovertebral veins, 73
Children and adolescents
 astrocytoma, 23, 25
 cerebellar hemisphere tumors, 23, 25
  cystic astrocytoma, 23
 fourth ventricle tumors, 24, 129
  choroid plexus papilloma, 25–26
  ependymona, 24
  medulloblastomas, 23–24, 129
 posterior fossa tumors, 23–25
 vertebral angiographic techniques, 4–5
  injection of contrast material, 7–8
Cholesteatomas, primary and secondary, 92
Chondromas of skull base, 92
 prepontine tumors, 94
Chordomas, 91, 92, 94, 100
 clival, 93–94, *101*
Choroid arch, 42–43
 posterior displacement, 121
 twigs to choroid plexus of fourth ventricle, 46–47
 vermian and hemispheric tumors, 147, *153*
Choroid plexus, *56, 58*
 and superior choroidal veins, 85
Choroid plexus papilloma, 91, 129, 134
 childhood tumor, 25–26
 pathology, 25–26
Choroidal arteries, posterior, 68–69
Choroidal branches of PICA
 fourth ventricle tumors, 134, *136*
Choroidal loop
 vermian and hemispheric tumors, 154
Choroidal point, 43, *44*, 46, *56, 58,* 122
 inferior vermian tumors, 146
 PICA, *41*
Choroidal veins, choroid plexus and superior
  choroidal veins, 85
Choroidal vessels
 quadrigeminal plate tumors, 124
 vermian and hemispheric tumors, 154, 163–165, *173, 174*
Chromophobe adenomas, 100
Cisterna magna, 24
 fourth ventricle tumors, 134, *135, 136,* 138
Circulation, posterior fossa, 1
 methods of opacification, 1–2
Cisterns, 20
Clival arteries, meningiomas, 92, 94, *98, 99, 100*
 blood supply, 94–95
 hypertrophied dorsal clival artery, 94, *99*
Clival chordomas, *101*
Clivus, 26
 fourth ventricle tumors, 137, *142, 143, 144*
 intracranial meningiomas, 92
Cochlear end organ, 21
Colliculo-central angle, 121
 quadrigeminal plate tumors, *124*
Colliculo-central point, 122
 measurement for position of 82*n*
Communicating artery
 arterior, 65*n*
 posterior, 37, 67
Complications of vertebral angiography, 9–11
Condyloid foramen, anterior (hypoglossal canal), 48
Conray 60 (meglumine iothalamate), 7
Contrast material
 direct injection into subclavian artery, 1
 radiopaque, 1, 7–8
 reflux into subclavian artery, 1
 test injection, 7
 toxic effects, 10
 vertebral angiography, 7–8
Copular points, *41, 44,* 47, 54
 fourth ventricle tumors, *34*–35, 131, 134
 inferior vermian tumors, *118,* 121, 146–147, *149, 152*
 of inferior vermian vein, *118,* 121, 122
 measurement of 47*n*
 normal anatomy, 53
Cortical branches of posterior cerebral arteries, 65
Cranial loop, 43
 or choroid arch, 42–43
Cranial nerve tumors, clinical aspects, 21–22
 neurinomas of fifth, seventh, tenth, and

twelfth nerve, 91
neurinomas of ninth, tenth, or eleventh nerve, 105, *109*
Craniectomy, midline suboccipital, 27
Craniopharyngiomas, 100
Crural-interdepuncular segment, 43
Culmen, 63–64

Demerol (meperidine hydrochloride), 5
Dermoid cysts, 106
Diabetes, insipidus, 22
Diagnosis of posterior fossa tumors, 176–179
   angioarchitecture of tumors, 176
   bone erosion, 176
   bone thinning, 176
   calcification, 176
   fifth nerve neurinomas, 178
   glomus jugulare tumors, 178
   hemangioblastomas, 178
   hyperostosis, 176
   location of tumor, 176
   meningiomas, 177–178
   miscellaneous tumors, 179
   patient's age and, 176
   soft tissue densities, 176
Dorsal clival artery, clival meningiomas and, 94, *99*, 100
Dorsal meningeal artery, 72, *99*
Dorsum sellae, *96*
Dura matter, 71, 100

Embolizations, catheter manipulation and, 10–11
Ependymomas, 91, 129, 134, *141*, 163, 179
   childhood tumor, 24
   fourth ventricle, 131, *132*, *133*
   pathology, 24
   surgical considerations, 27
Epidermoids, 91–92
   angiographic changes, 105–106
   in cerebellopontine angle, 92
Epidural veins, cervical, 75
Extra-axial tumor, 26, 91, 157–160
   acoustic neurinomas, 26
   meningiomas, 26, 158, 160
   pneumoencephalography for evaluating, 28
   retrocerebellar, 106
   tentorial, 157–160
Eyes, tumor affecting, 21–22

Femoral artery, percutaneous puncture and catheter insertion, 1–2
Femoral puncture
   complications, 9–10
Fibromas, 106
Fifth nerve neurinomas, differential diagnosis, 91, 101, 178
Foramina, fourth ventricle tumors, 134
Foramen magnum, 31, 36, 71
   angiographic anatomy, 49, *52*
   meningiomas, 26, 92
   surgical considerations, 27
   tonsillar herniation, 151, *155*, *156*, *159*
Foramen transversarium, 31
Fourth ventricle tumors, 21, 24–25, *34–35*
   angiographic features, *34–35*, 46
   anterior displacements, 129–131
   children and adolescents, 24–25, 129
   choroid plexus, papilloma, 25–26, *56*, *58*
   cisterna magna tumor mass and, *134*, *135*, *136*, *138*
   clinical aspects, 21
   colored plate diagram, *34–35*
   differential diagnosis from pontine tumors, 116, *120*, 134, *136*, *139*, *145*, 177
   ependymoma, 24, *56*, *58*
   lateral displacements, 132–137
   measurements for evaluating position of choroidal point and vessels, 46n
   meningiomas, 177
   pathology, 24–25
   posterior displacement, 131–132
   superior displacement, 131
   surgical considerations, 28
   Twining's point for, 46, 82n, 122
   vein of lateral recess. *See* Vein of lateral recess of fourth ventricle
   vermian and hemispheric tumors, 147

Geniculate body arteries, 67–68
Glial tumors, 115
Glioblastomas multiforme, 115
   diagnosis, 179
Gliomas, 91, 163
   brainstem tumors, 115, 122
   eccentric, 122–123
   optic nerve, 91
   prepontine and cerebellopontine angle cisterns, 91
   quadrigeminal plate tumors, 123–*124*
Glomus jugulare tumors, 91, 94, 104, 165

Index

Glomus jugulare tumors *(continued)*
　angiographic appearance, 104–105, 178
　arteriovenous shunts and, 176
　blood supply from ascending pharyngeal artery, 178
　differential diagnosis, 178
　vascular displacement, 104–105
Great vein of Galen, *64*
　aneurysms of, 165

Headaches, 23
Hemangioblastomas, 26, 163
　angiographic appearances, *158, 159,* 178
　blood supply, 178
　cerebellar, 165
　cerebellar hemispheric, *158*
　cyst and nodule, 26
　differential diagnosis, 178
　　arteriovenous malformation, *148, 149,* 178
　pathology, 26
Hematoma formation, 9
Hemiparesis, 11
Hemispheric arteries
　angiographic anatomy, 62, 63
Hemispheric branches of PICA, *56*
Hemispheric tumors. *See also* Vermian and hemispheric tumors
　inferior, *34–35,* 146–151
　　angiographic anatomy, *34–35*
　superior, *34–35*
　　angiographic anatomy, *34–35*
Hemispheric veins, 83–84
　superior and inferior, 76
　superior vermian and superior hemispheric tumors, 153–166
Hemorrhages, pontine, 123
Heparinization of patient, 10
Heparinized-saline perfusion, 7
Hippocampal gyrus, 65
Hydrocephalus
　CSF obstruction and, 21–22
　communicating, 137, *142*
　fourth ventricle tumors, 137
　hemangioblastomas and, 26
　rise in intracranial pressure and, 21, 22
　shunts prior to surgery, 29
　surgical considerations, 27, 29
　ventriculography, 28
Hyperostosis and diagnosis of posterior fossa tumors, 176

Hypertension, intracranial, 22
Hypertrophy, pontine, 25
Hypoglossal arteries, 48, 70
Hypophyseal artery, inferior, 72

Inferior cerebellar arteries, normal anatomy, *32–33*
Inferior cerebellar hemisphere, inferior vermian and hemispheric tumors, 147
Inferior hemispheric vein, *34–35*
　inferior hemispheric tumors, 146–151, *154, 157*
　angiographic anatomy, *34–35*
Inferior hypophyseal artery, 72
Inferior vermian arteries and veins
　angiographic anatomy, *34–35, 55, 77, 78, 79, 81, 82, 83,* 122
　variations, 87
　copular point, *118,* 121, 146–147, *149, 152*
　fourth ventricle tumors, 134, *140*
　vermian and hemispheric tumors, 154
Inferior vermian hemangioblastoma, *149*
Inferior vermian segments of PICA, *44, 58*
Inferior vermian tumors, 146–151, *153*
　angiographic anatomy, *34–35,* 87
　involving inferior cerebellar hemisphere, 147
　involving vermis, 146–147
　midline position, 147, *148, 150, 152*
Infratentorial meningiomas, 177
Infratonsillar segments, 50, *56, 57,* 60
　medial, *57, 60*
Internal auditory artery. *See also* Labyrinthine artery
　angiographic anatomy, 61–62
　stretching and displacement, 100
　tumor stains, 176
Internal auditory canal, 55
　AICA, *61*
Internal carotid artery, 37, 65n
　angiography, 105, 163
　meningohypophyseal branch, *99, 100, 112, 172,* 178
Internal cerebral vein, 85
Interpeduncular cistern, *44, 49,* 64–65
Interpeduncular-crural segment, 62–63
Intracranial pressure syndrome, 21–22
Infratentorial tumors, diagnosis, 178

Jugular vein, 73, *74*
　glomus jugulare tumors, 104

Kidney, metastatic tumors to cerebellum
   originating in, 179

Labyrinthine artery (internal auditory artery)
   angiographic anatomy, 61–62
   displacement, 100
   tumor stain, 176
Lethargy, symptoms of, 22

Magnification techniques, 11
Marginal artery, 62
   angiographic anatomy, 62
Mastoid infection and sinus thrombosis, 165
Medulla, *43, 60*
Medulla oblongata, 40
Medullary arteries, 40
Medullary segments of PICA, *50, 56, 57, 58, 60*
Medullary tumors, 35
   on posterior inferior cerebellar arteries, *35*
Medulloblastomas, 129
   cerebellar vermis, site of, 23–24
   children and adolescents, 23–24, *138, 139, 140*
   diagnosis, *138*, 179
   fourth ventricle tumors and, 134
   involving nodulus, *138, 147*
   pathology, 23–24
   surgical considerations, 27
Meningeal arteries, 48
   angiographic anatomy, 71–73
   anterior branch, *39*, 71, *97*
      prepontine tumors, *94, 95*
   anterosuperior group, 71–72
   dorsal, 72, *99*
   inferior group, 71
   inferior hypophyseal artery, 72
   lateral group, 72
   meningeal branches of ascending pharyngeal artery, 73, *98*
   meningeal branches of external carotid artery, 104
   meningeal branches of external occipital artery, 72, *170*
   middle, 72
      clival meningiomas, 95, *170*
      posterior branch, 72, *170*
      recurrent branches, 72
   normal anatomy, 71–73
   posterior branch, *53*, 71, *110, 111, 162, 164*
   tentorial artery, 72

vermian and hemispheric tumors, 165, *170, 171*
Meningiomas, 21, 28, 91–92
   basilar artery displacement, 104, *110, 111, 112*
   blood supply, 177
      from meningohypophyseal branch of internal carotid artery, *99, 100, 112, 172,* 178
   cerebellar convexity, 92, 177–178
   cerebellopontine angle, 104, *110, 111, 112*
   clinical aspects, 21
   clival, 94–95, *98, 99, 100*
      blood supply, 94–95
   differential diagnosis, 177–178
      fourth ventricle meningiomas, 177
      infratentorial meningiomas, 177
      supratentorial meningiomas, 177
      tumor stains, *98, 170, 171, 175,* 176–177
      vascular stains, 177
   extra-axial tumors, 26, 158, 160
   meningeal branch of vertebral artery, 165, *174*
   pathology, 26
   in posterior fossa, 92
   prepontine and cerebellopontine angle tumors, 91
   supratentorial, 177
   tentorial, 162, 163, *172, 173, 174*
      burrowing into cerebellar hemisphere, *168, 170, 171*
Meningohypophyseal artery, 105
Meningohypophyseal branch of internal carotid artery
   blood supply to meningiomas, *99, 100, 112, 172,* 178
Meningohypophyseal trunk, 71
Mesencephalic vein
   anatomy, *34*–35
   displacement with midbrain tumor, 120
   fifth cranial nerve neurinomas, 101
   fourth ventricle tumors, 134
   midbrain tumors, 119, *120*
   posterior, 64, 79–81
   quadrigeminal plate tumors, *121*, 124, *126, 127*
Mesencephalon, 63
Metastatic tumors, 25, 163
   to cerebellum, 179
   to lower clivus, 94
   to petrous bone, 91

Index

Methyl glucamine compounds, 11
Microscope, operating, 29
Midbrain tumors, 35
   colored plate diagram, *34*
   intra-axial, 163
   superior cerebellar artery, *119*
Midline suboccipital craniectomy, surgical exposures, 27
Midpointine tumor, 35
   angiographic anatomy, 35
   colored plate diagram, *34–35*
Mucoceles of sphenoid sinus, 91

Needles and catheters, 1
Nembutal (sodium pentobarbitol), 4
Neurinomas
   acoustic. *See* Acoustic neurinomas
   fifth nerve, 101, 178
   of fifth, seventh, tenth, and twelfth cranial nerves, 91
   ninth, tenth, or eleventh cranial nerves, 105, *109*
Neurofibromatosis of van Recklinghausen's disease, 91–92
Neurological deficits, following vertebral angiography, 10–11
   posterior fossa tumors, 20
Neuroradiology suite, preparation of patient, 4
Nodulus, *43, 53, 56*
   hypertrophy, 118
   medulloblastomas involving, *138*, 147
   from supratonsillar segment of PICA, *138*, 179
Nystagmus, 25

Occipital artery, 38
   internal, *44, 45, 58, 59*, 66
   meningeal branch of external, 72, *170*
   vermian and hemispheric tumors, 165, *170*
Occipital branch of posterior cerebral artery, *63*
Occipital lobe, *44, 45, 59*, 65, 66
Occipital squamosa, *158*
Occipital veins, 85
Occipitovertebral anastomosis, 48
Oliogodendrogliomas or metastases, 115
   of cerebellar tonsil, *158*
Optic nerve gliomas, 91
Otic artery, 70

Palsy, sixth nerve, 22
Papilledema, 21, 22, 29
   clinical aspects, 21–22

Papillomas, choroid plexus, 129, 134
Paraplegia, 11
Paresis, 21
Parieto-occipital arteries, *14, 45, 58, 59*, 66–67
Parinaud's syndrome, 22
Pathology, posterior fossa tumors, 22–26
Patients, explaining angiographic technique to, 4
Pericallosal artery, posterior, 67, *68*
Persistent trigeminal artery, 70
Petrosal vein
   angiographic anatomy, 77–78, *79, 81, 82, 87*
   variations, 86
   cerebellopontine angle tumors, 100–101, *104, 105, 106*
Petrous bone
   meningiomas, 26, 92
   metastatic tumors, 91
   rhabdomyosarcoma, 165
Pharyngeal artery. *See* Ascending pharyngeal artery
Phenergan (promethazine hydrochloride), 5
PICA. *See* Posterior inferior cerebellar artery
Pineal gland, 124
Pineal region tumors, 21–22, 123, 165
   clinical aspects, 21–22
   surgical considerations, 29
Pituitary adenomas, 91
Plasmocytomas, 94
Pneumoencephalography, 134
   angiography and, 27–28
Polycythemia and hemangioblastomas, 26
Pons
   angiographic signs of expansion, 115
   anterior displacements, 115–118
   lower, *43, 55*
   superior cerebellar artery, *64*
   upper, *43, 64*
Pontine arteries
   angiographic anatomy, 61
   hypertrophy, 25
   lateral displacements, *119, 121*
   normal anatomy, *34–35*, 61, *117, 121*
   pontine and mesencephalic tumors, *117*
Pontine glioma, 115–120, *117, 118, 119, 120, 121*
   exophytic extension into cerebellopontine angle cistern, 120
   with major involvement of medulla, *122*

Pontine tegmentum, 21
Pontine tumors, *117*, 157
  anatomy, *34*–35
  angiographic signs of pontine expansion, 115
    anterior displacements, 115–116, *117, 118*
    lateral displacements, 118,*119, 120, 121, 128*
    posterior displacements, *117, 118, 119, 120, 121, 122, 123*
  colored plate diagram, *34*
  differential diagnosis of pontine from fourth ventricle tumors, 115–120, 134, *136, 139, 145*
    position of lateral recess of the fourth ventricle, *120*
  normal anatomy, *34*–35, 61, *117, 121*
  quadrigeminal plate tumors, *121*, 123, *124, 125, 126*
Pontomedullary cistern, fourth ventricle tumors, 134
Pontomedullary junction, *55*
Ponto-mesencephalic vein, 76
  angiographic anatomy, 76
    variations, 85–86
  angiographic displacement, *96*
  angiotomography of, 18
  anterior, 18
  brainstem tumors, 122
  fifth cranial nerve neurinomas, 101
  fourth ventricle tumors, 131,*132, 136*, 137, *142, 143, 144*
  inferior vermian tumors, 146
  midbrain tumors, *118*
  pontine and mesencephalic tumors, 115–118
  pontine segment displacement and fourth ventricle tumors, 131, *132, 136*
  prepontine tumors and displacement of, 93, 96
  vermian and hemispheric tumors, 154
Posterior branch of middle meningeal artery, 72, *170*
Posterior cerebral arteries, 44
  angiographic anatomy, *37, 38*, 64–69
    variations, 69–70
  anterior temporal artery, 65
  calcarine branch, *45*, 66–67
  cerebellopontine angle tumors, *97*, 101, *103, 109, 111*
  cortical branches, 65
  occipital branch, *63*
  parieto-occipital and calcarine arteries, 66–67
  penetrating branches, 67
  pontine and mesencephalic tumors, 119–120
  posterior choroidal arteries, 68–69
  posterior pericallosal artery, 67
  posterior temporal artery, *45*, 65–66
  quadrigeminal and geniculate body arteries, 67–68, 157, *166*
  separation of superior cerebellar arteries and, 157
  thalamoperforating arteries, 67
  vermian and hemispheric tumors, 163, *173*
Posterior choroidal arteries, *68, 69, 70*
Posterior communicating artery, 67*n*, 68
Posterior fossa
  angiographic anatomy, 31–90
    basilar artery, 52–70
    meningeal arteries, 71–73
    veins, 73–87
      variations, 85–87
    vertebral artery, 31–52
      variations, 47–52
  circulation, 1
  meningiomas, 92
  opacification, 1
  surgical considerations, 26–27
  veins
    angiographic anatomy, 75–84
    anterior (petrosal) group, 75–76
    brachial veins, 76
    cerebellomedullary vein, 77
    inferior vermian vein, 84
    petrosal vein, 77–79
    ponto-mesencephalic vein, 76
    posterior mesencephalic veins, 79–81
    posterior (tentorial) group, 83
    precentral cerebellar vein, 81–83
    superior and inferior hemispheric veins, 76
    superior (Galenic) group, 79
    superior vermian vein, 83
    vein of lateral recess of fourth ventricle, 76–77
  venous drainage, 73–75
Posterior fossa tumors. *See also specific tumors*
  adult tumors, 25–26
  arterial displacements, 46
  childhood tumors, 23–25
  differential diagnosis, 176–179

Posterior fossa tumors *(continued)*
  pathology, 22–26
    adult tumors, 25–26
    childhood tumors, 23–25
  surgical considerations, 26–28
  syndromes, 20–22
    general involvement, 22
    regional involvement, 20–22
Posterior inferior cerebellar artery (PICA), 24–25, 40–47, 53
  angiographic anatomy, 32–33, 40, *41, 42, 43, 44,* 45, 46–47
  variations, 47–52, 69–70
  angiographic feature of fourth ventricle tumors, 46
  anterior medullary segment, 40–45, *45*
  caudal and cranial loops, 40–43, 49, 52, *92,* 102
    tonsillar herniation, *52,* 151
  cerebellopontine angle tumors, *92,* 102
  choroidal branches, fourth ventricle tumors, 134, *136*
  choroidal points, *34–35, 41,* 116
  cranial loop or choroid arch, 42–43
  differential diagnosis of pontine from fourth ventricle tumors, 116, *120,* 134, *136,* 139, *145,* 177
  ependymoma, 24
  evaluation of position of choroidal point and vessels, 46*n*
  fourth ventricle tumors, 131
    colored plate diagram, *34*
  hemispheric branches, *56*
  inferior hemispheriic and vermian branches, *41*
    inferior vermian and inferior hemispheric tumors, 147, *155, 156, 161*
  infratonsillar segment, 50, *56, 57,* 60
  lateral medullary segment, 45, 116
  lateral supratonsillar segment, 49, *54,* 55
  loops, *50–51*
  low pontine tumor, *128*
  medial supratonsillar segment, 49, *53, 55, 58, 59*
  medullary segments, *57, 58,* 60
  nodular branches, hypertrophy and posterior displacement, 147
  normal anatomy, *41, 42, 43, 44, 45*
  point of origin and course, 40, *41, 42*
  pontine and mesencephalic tumors
    lateral dissplacements, 118–119, *120, 128*
  posterior displacements, 117, 120–121, *122,* 123
  pontine glioma, *122*
  posterior medullary segment, 40, 45, *50, 56, 57, 58,* 60, 116
    fourth ventricle tumors, *130,* 131, *133, 135*
  retrotonsillar segment, *35, 41, 43, 44, 56,* 116
    fourth ventricle tumors, *130,* 131, *135*
    inferior vermian tumors, 146
  Sahlstedt's point for the aqueduct, 46
  superior retrotonsillar segment, 47
  superior vermian and hemispheric tumors, 156, *161*
  supratonsillar segments, *34–35, 41, 42, 43, 50,* 53, 54, *55, 57, 58,* 116
    fourth ventricle tumors, *130,* 131, 132, *133, 135, 138, 145*
    inferior vermian tumors, 146, 148, 149, 150
    nodular vessels derived from, *138,* 179
    vermian and hemispheric tumors, 147, *153*
  surgical considerations, 28
  tonsillohemispheric branch, *43, 44,* 47, 50, *56, 58, 59,* 155
  Twining's point for fourth ventricle, 46, 82*n,* 122
  vermian and hemispheric tumors, 147, 149–151, *153,* 154, *158*
Posterior ullary segments, 40, 45, *50, 56, 57, 58,* 60, 116
Posterior meningeal branch, 53
Posterioor mesencephalic vein, 64, 79–81
Posterior pericallosal artery, 67, *68*
Poststerior spinal artery, 40
Posterior temporal artery, *44, 45, 58, 59,* 65–66
Precentral cerebellar artery
  posterior displacement, *117, 118,* 121
Precentral cerebellar vein, *64, 77,* 81–82, *83*
  angiographic anatomy, *64,* 81–83
  variations, 86–87
  angiotomography, 18
  brainstem tumors, 122
  deformities and displacement of colliculo-central point, 82
  differential diagnosis of pontine from fourth ventricle tumors, 116
  fourth ventricle tumors, *34–35,* 131, *132,* 134, *143*

Precentral cerebellar vein *(continued)*
  hemispheric astrocytoma, *166, 167*
  posterior displacement, 121
  quadrigeminal plate tumors, 124, *125*
  vermian and hemispheric tumors, *118, 154, 157, 161, 164, 167*
Precentral lobule of cerebellum, 43, *64*
Prepontine tumors, 93–97
  angiographic anatomy, *32–33, 92, 93, 94, 95, 96, 101*
  basilar artery displacement, *92, 93, 94, 95*
  color plate diagrams, *33*
  common, 91
  hypertrophied dorsal clival arteries, 94, *99*
  rare lesions, 91
Pressure, syndrome of raised intracranial pressure, 21–22
Pro-atlantal intersegmental artery, 48
Pseudoaneurysm formation, 10
Puberty, precocious, 22
Pyramis, 43, *53*

Quadrigeminal artery, 43, 67–68
Quadrigeminal cistern, 43
Quadrigeminal plate tumors, *121*, 123, *124, 125, 126, 127*

Radial artery, 1
Radiographic studies
  evaluation of preoperative, 27–28
  tumor's location and size, 27
Radiographic techniques
  subtraction, 11–18
  vertebral angiography, 11
Radiopaque contrast material, 1, 7–8
Raised intracranial pressure, 21–22, 28
  etiology of, 22
Renografin 60 (meglumine diatrizoate), 7–8
Retrocerebellar extra-axial tumors, 106
Retrotonsillar branches of PICA, *34–35, 41, 43, 44, 56, 58*
  fourth ventricle tumors, *130*, 131, *135*
Rhabdomyosarcoma, originating from petrous bone, 165

Saline perfusion solution, 7
Secobarbital, 5
Sedation, angiographic technique, 4–5
  infants and children, 5
Seldinger technique, 1–2, 5
Sinuses, 91
  vermian and hemispheric tumors, 165–166, *175*

Sixth nerve palsy, 22
Sphenoid sinus, mucoceles of, 91
Spinal arteries
  anterior, *37, 39, 51*
    angiographic anatomy, 51
    pontine and mesencephalic tumors, 118
  posterior, 40
Spinal cord, veins, 75
Stains
  oblique frontal projection, 177
  tumor
    acoustic neurinomas, *106, 107*, 176–177
    astrocytomas, 179
    hemangioblastomas, 178
    meningiomas, *98, 170, 171, 175*, 176–177
  vascular, 176, 177
Subarachnoid spaces, pneumoencephalography for evaluating, 28
Subclavian angiography, 8, 38
  catheterization, 1–2
  fluoroscopic visualization, 10
  injections of contrast material, 1
  percutaneous angiography, 1
Suboccipital craniectomy, 27
Suboccipital venous plexus, 74–75
Subtraction technique, 11–18
  diapositive prints, 11
  masks, 12
  methods and films used, 12–18
    first order subtraction, 12–15
    second order subtraction, 15–18
Superior cerebellar artery, 43, 62–64
  ambient, 116
  ambient segments, *58, 59, 64*, 116
  angiographic anatomy, 32, 62–64
  variations, 70
  colored plate diagram, *33*
  branches, *57, 58, 62, 63, 64*
  cerebellopontine angle tumors, 97, 101, *103, 109, 111*
  crural segment, *44, 58, 59, 64*
  differential diagnosis of pontine from fourth ventricle tumors, 116
  hemispheric arteries, 62
  hemispheric astrocytoma, *166, 167*
  hemispheric branches, 58, 63, 160
    vermian and hemispheric tumors, 160–162, *168*
  interpeduncular-crural segment, *43, 44, 49,*

Index

Superior cerebellar artery *(continued)*
    58, 59, 62–63
  marginal branch, *57,* 62
  midbrain tumors, *119*
  quadrigeminal plate tumors, *121, 124, 125, 126*
  quadrigeminal segments, *58, 59, 64*
  segments, *43, 44, 58, 59,* 62, *64*
  site of origin, *43, 44, 45, 49, 58,* 62
  superior vermian artery, 62–64, 116
    fourth ventricle tumors, *130,* 131, *132, 135*
    vermian and hemispheric tumors, *150, 154,* 157, *160, 162, 164, 166*
Superior hemispheric tumors. *See also* Vermian and hemispheric tumors
  anatomy, *34–35*
Superior vermian artery, 43
  angiographic anatomy, 62–64
  interpeduncular-crural segment, 62–63
Superior vermian tumors, 153–166. *See also* Vermian and hemispheric tumors
  anatomy, *34–35*
Supratentorial meningiomas, 177
Supratentorial veins, 84–87
Supratonsillar segments of PICA *34–35, 41, 42–43, 50, 53, 54, 55, 58,* 116
Surgical considerations, 26–28
  innovations, 29
  operating microscopes, 29
  posterior fossa tumors, 26–28
    exploration and resection, 27
    innovation, 29
    preoperative evaluation, 27–28
    routine exposures, 27
  shunts prior to surgery, 29
  techniques of evaluation, 27–28
Sylvian aqueduct, 20

Temporal artery
  anterior, *59,* 65, *66*
  posterior, *44, 45, 58, 59,* 65–66
Tentorial artery, 72, *172*
  course of, 163
  hemangioblastomas, 178
  vermian and hemispheric tumors, 162, *172*
Tentorial incisura, 71
Tentorium, 63
  extra-axial tumors, 157–160
  meningiomas, 92, 162, 163, *172*
    burrowing into cerebellar hemisphere, *168, 170, 171*
    originating from posterior lip of tentorium, 162, *172, 173, 174*
Thalamic region, tumors, 29
Thalamic veins, 85
Thalamoperforating arteries, anterior and posterior, 67, *68, 69*
Third cervical spinal nerve root, 38
Third cervical vertebra, 31
Third ventricle
  dilatation of anterior, 91
  tumors, 29
Thorazine (chlorpromazine), 5
Thromboembolism, complication of vertebral angiography, 9
Thrombosis, with ischemia of lower leg, 9
Thyrocervical trunk, *51*
Thyroid gland tumors, 179
Tonsils, *43, 53, 56*
  cerebellar tonsil tumors, 147–151
  relationship of PICA to, 49
Tonsillar herniation, 27, 49, 151, *155, 156*
  evaluation of, 11
  surgical considerations, 27
Tonsillohemispheric artery, 151, *156*
Tonsillohemispheric branch of PICA, *43, 44, 47, 50, 56, 58, 59, 155*
Transverse myelitis, 11
Transverse pontine veins, 122–123
  posterior displacement, *96*
Trigeminal artery, persistent, 70
Trigeminal ganglia, 72
Trigeminal neurinomas, 100, 163
Tumor stains
  acoustic neurinomas, *106, 107,* 176–177
  meningiomas, *98, 170, 171, 175,* 176–177
Tumors. *See also specific tumors*
  acoustic neurinomas, 21, 26
  adult, 25–26
    acoustic neurinomas, 26
    cerebellum, 26
    extra-axial masses, 26
    hemangioblastomas, 26
    meningiomas, 26
    blockage of CSF pathways, 22
  brainstem, 25
  cerebellopontine angle, 28, 32–33
  cerebellum, hemangioblastomas, 26
  childhood, 23–25
    astrocytoma, 23, 25
    brainstem, 25

Tumors *(continued)*
  cerebellar hemisphere, 23
  cerebellar vermis, 23–24
  choroid plexus papilloma, 24–25
  ependymoma, 24
  fourth ventricle, 24–25
  medulloblastoma, 23–24
  clinical aspects, 20–22
  diagnostic evaluation, 27–29
  extra-axial, 26, 28
  fourth ventricle, 24–25, 35
  hemangioblastoma, 25–26
  histologic nature, 27
  inferior hemispheric, *34–35*
  inferior vermian, *34–35*
  medullary, *34–35*
  meningiomas, 26
  mesencephalic, 35
  midbrain, 35
  midpontine, 35
  neurological syndromes, 20
  pathology, 22–26
    adult tumors, 25–26
    childhood tumors, 23–25
  pontine, 35
  prepontine and cerebellopontine angle, 32–33, 91–117
    color plate diagrams, *33*
  raised intracranial pressure, 22
  rapidity of growth, 20
  regional involvement, 20–22
    brainstem, 21
    cerebellopontine angle, 21
    cerebellum, 20–21
    fourth ventricle, 21
    pineal region, 21–22
    size and location, techniques of evaluation, 27–28
  superior hemispheric, *34–35*
  superior vermian, *34–35*
  supratentorial, 26
  surgical considerations, 26–28
    angiography for diagnostic evaluation, 29
    brainstem gliomas, 29
    cerebellopontine angle, 28
    fourth ventricle, 28
    operating microscope, 29
    pineal region, 29
    preoperative evaluation, 27–28
    shunts to relieve hydrocephalus, 29
    techniques of evaluation, 27–28

Twining's line, 46, 82*n*, 122
Tympanum, glomus jugulare tumors, 104

Uvula, *43*

Valium (diazepam), 4
van Recklinghausen's disease, neurofibromatosis of, 91–92
Vein of the lateral recess of fourth ventricle, *55*
  cerebellar hemispheric hemangioblastoma, *158*
  fourth ventricle tumors, 134, *136, 139, 145*
    differential diagnosis of pontine glioma from fourth ventricle tumor, 116, *120*, 134, *136, 139, 145*
  low pontine tumor, *128*
  vermian and hemispheric tumors, 147, *154*
Veins. *See also specific veins*
  angiographic anatomy, 73–87
  basal vein of Rosenthal, 84–85
  cervical epidural venous system, 75
  cervicovertebral, 73–75
  great vein of Galen, 77, *78,* 79
  hemispheric, 100
  jugular, 73, *74*
  mesencephalic, 100
  posterior fossa, 75–84
    anterior (petrosal) group, 75–76
    brachial veins, 76, *77, 78,* 79
    cerebellomedullary vein, 77
    inferior vermian vein, 77, *78, 79, 81, 82, 83, 84*
    petrosal vein, 77–78, *79, 81, 82,* 87
    ponto-mesencephalic vein, 76, *77, 78*
    posterior (tentorial) group, 83
    posterior mesencephalic veins, *77, 78, 79,* 80–81
    precentral cerebellar vein, 77, 81–82, *83*
    superior (Galenic) group, 79–81
    superior and inferior hemispheric veins, 76, *77, 78, 79,* 81
    superior vermian vein, *77, 78,* 83, *86*
    vein of lateral recess of fourth ventricle, 76–77, *80, 81, 82,* 100, *116*
  spinal cord, 75
  suboccipital venous plexus, *74–*75
  supratentorial, 84–87
    basal vein of Rosenthal, 84–85
    choroid plexus and superior choroidal veins, 85

Index

Veins *(continued)*
  internal cerebral vein, 85
    occipital veins, 85
    thalamic veins, 85
    variations, 85–87
  transverse pontine, 100
  vertebral, 73–74
Ventriculography, 134
  angiography and, 27–28
  pantopaque, 28
  role of, 27–28
Vermian and hemispheric tumors
  colored plate diagrams, *34*
    cystic astrocytoma, 151, *152*
  inferior, 146–151
    cerebellar tonsil tumor, 147–151
    colored plate diagrams, *34*
  superior, 153–166
    colored plate diagrams, *34*
  tonsillar herniation, 151–153
Vermian arteries
  inferior. *See* Inferior vermian artery
  superior. *See* Superior vermian artery
Vermian tumors
  inferior, *35*
  superior, *35*, 153–166
    angiographic anatomy, *35*
Vermian vein
  inferior, 84. *See also* Inferior vermian arteries and veins
  superior, 83. *See also* Superior vermian arteries
Vermis
  clinical aspects, 20–21
  fourth ventricle tumors, 134, *138*
  inferior vermian vein, 84
  quadrigeminal plate tumors, 124
  superior vermian vein, 83
  vermian and hemispheric tumors, 146
Vertebral angiographic technique, 4–19
  acoustic neurinomas, 104
  angiotomography, 18
  brachial angiography, 2, 8
  catheterization and catheters, 5–7
    dosage schedule for children, 5
    needle and catheter dimensions for different age groups, 6
  children and infants, 4–5
  complications, 9–11
    bleeding and thromboembolism, 9
    hematoma formation, 9
    local causes, 9
    manipulative causes, 9, 10–11
    neurological deficits, 10–11
    dosage schedule, 5, 7–8
    withdrawal of catheter, 7
  direct percutaneous brachial angiography, 2
  direct vertebral puncture, 1
  explaining to patient, 4
  guide wires, 5–7, 10
  heparinized-saline perfusion, 7
  historical development, 1–3
  opacification of posterior fossa, 1
  percutaneous retrograde brachial angiography, 2
  radiographic technique, 11
  routine procedure, 4
  sedation and local anesthesia for patient, 4–5
    dosage schedule for children, 5
  Seldinger's method, 1–2
  subclavian angiography, 8
  subtraction technique, 11–18
    first order subtractions, 12, *13, 14, 15*
    second order subtractions, 15–18, *16, 17, 18*
  supratentorial structures, 84
  technique of percutaneous puncture, 1–2
  transaxillary catheterization of vertebral artery, 2
Vertebral artery
  aneurysms, 91
  angiographic anatomy, 31–52, *32–33, 36*
    cervical branches, 38
    hypoplastic left vertebral artery, *57*
    intracranial branches, 38
    medullary arteries, 40
    meningeal arteries, 38, 71–73
    muscular branches, *37, 38, 39*
    posterior inferior cerebellar artery, 40–47
    supratonsillar segment, 53
    variations, 47–52, 70
      absent or hypoplastic (PICA), 48, *49, 50*
      site of origin, 47–48
  anterior meningeal branch, *94, 95*
  bifid anomaly of left vertebral artery, *140*
  catheterization, 2, 5
  cervical branches, 38
  colored plate diagrams, *33*
  direct puncture, 1
  fluoroscopic assessment, 5
  left, 36

Vertebral artery *(continued)*
  muscular branches, 38
  opacifying methods, 1
  percutaneous puncture, 1
    complications following, 10
  spinal artery, 38–40
    anterior, *37, 39, 51*
    posterior, 40
  transaxillary catheterization, 2
  urethral catheter injection, 1
Vertebral veins, 73–74
Visual loss, 22
Vomiting, 21, 22, 25